ROBIN M. GRAY R.N.

BREAST LUMP
WHAT LIES BENEATH?

A Must Read Memoir And Guide
That May Help Others Avoid the Common
Pitfalls of a Doctor Related Breast Cancer
Misdiagnosis

Sonshine Publishing
United States of America

BREAST LUMP WHAT LIES BENEATH
ROBIN M. GRAY R.N.

Copyright 2009 by Robin M. Gray R.N.
Version 1.1
Sonshine Publishing
United States of America

IBSN: 978-0-615-23514-1
Library of Congress Control Number: 2008907503

Contributing Physicians: I appreciate Dr. William H. Goodson III, M.D., top breast surgeon, and Dr. Orlando E. Silva, M.D., a top medical oncologist, for their personal contacts of encouragement to me and for their contributions made in this book.
Book Cover Designers: Angi Shearstone and Robin M. Gray
Editing: Quadrant Infotech (India)

Author Online
    You may visit Robin M. Gray's book website for updates and information.

For Further Help
    Although the author is glad to receive feedback, she cannot provide private consultation on publishing material. For further help, please see the bibliography and web site resources listed at the end of this book.

Dedicated to my most supportive and loving family, to young women who have breast lumps, to women who have suffered a breast cancer misdiagnosis, and to all who yearn to know the truth.

Contents

Preface

At thirty-eight years of age, I was smooth sailing through life until I discovered a lump in my breast. However, it was thoroughly assessed by my doctors, and I was repeatedly informed that I only had a benign fibrocystic breast condition. I had faith in my many well-respected physicians and the benign lab reports. Additionally, everything that I read about fibrocystic breast disease seemed to fit my breast lump and my surgeon's fibrocystic breast diagnosis. Nonetheless, I was about to experience one of the most medically mishandled cases that I have ever known. I would have never dreamed something like this could happen to me, a nurse, and my husband, a physician.

Seventeen months after I first saw my doctors for a breast lump, I was delayed diagnosed with breast cancer. Unfortunately, due to the late diagnosis, I suffered a worse prognosis that required many more treatments than if I had been immediately diagnosed.

After my misdiagnosis, I learned that numerous physician errors led to my delayed diagnosis. Additionally, I learned that because breast cancer is rarer in younger women, the risk of it being misdiagnosed is high. Sadly, I didn't learn the best-kept medical secret sooner.

However, I believe my story will help and educate other young women about breast lumps. In chapters one through three, my misdiagnosis is explained to point out some of the causes of a breast cancer misdiagnosis. In the postscript, I thoroughly explain causes and prevention of a breast cancer misdiagnosis.

I also believe my story will encourage those who have already suffered from the tragedy of a breast cancer misdiagnosis. The book has helpful tips on breast cancer treatments, on misdiagnosis litigation, and on emotional healing in chapters four through seven.

As you journey through my story, I trust you will be aided and enlightened. Should you learn and be saved some suffering after reading my story, some of my past sorrows will turn into joy.

Acknowledgements

I would like to acknowledge and thank my children and husband for their patience while I transformed my ambitions of writing about my misdiagnosis into a reality. I also thank my family, friends, and many physicians who have endlessly assisted and encouraged me. Additionally, I want to thank the heroes, women who have fought breast cancer, which I have had the privilege of being encouraged by. Last, but not least, I thank God, who has taught me survival through it all, and to truly love, forgive, and never give up, for each day is a precious gift from above.

Legal Disclaimers

In this book, the names of some healthcare providers and health care institutions/offices directly or remotely involved with my misdiagnosis have been changed in order to protect the identities of individuals and or businesses, and that any similarities to actual persons, either living or dead, are merely coincidental. In order to further protect identities, I have used my maiden name. While some names, character traits, and locations have been changed, the misdiagnosis story itself is truly presented in order to implicate a vital warning to all young women with breast lumps.

This book is intended to educate and should not be used as a replacement or alternative to appropriate medical or legal consultation. I have exerted every effort to ensure that the information presented is accurate, complete, and as up to date as possible at the time of publication. However, research and medicine is an ever-evolving process.

You acknowledge that the author, Robin Gray R.N, and agents are not engaged in the practice of medicine or law. This book is presented to enhance your knowledge and support the relationship that exists between you and your lawyer and/or physician. All decisions made using or relying on the legal and medical information provided by this book will be solely your responsibility, not Robin Gray R.N. and her agents.

<u>ROBIN GRAY R.N.</u>
BREAST LUMP
WHAT LIES BENEATH?

Chapter 1

Stormy Discovery

Physician delay in the diagnosis of breast cancer is common. In previous studies, 6-16 percent of women with breast cancer experienced physician–caused delay in diagnosis. Delay has been associated with younger patients...

_Archives of Internal Medicine, June 24, 2002

O n an overcast gray November afternoon in 2000, melancholic cold winds cried down an endless mountain of young autumn trees. Launched in the sky were thousands of brown necrotic leaves that blew about like birds lost in flight. When they finally landed, they were in the valley below where my home resided in rural upstate, New York.

Inside our brand new dream house, I was having fun playing hide and seek with my three young boys, ages two, seven, and nine years old, while my husband, Isaac, was busily reading the Sunday newspaper. After a long while of running merrily around the house with my kids, I was tired, so I plopped down into our sofa to relax.

After a few minutes of lounging, I figured a soothing bath would be just the thing that I needed to unwind and relax some more. Therefore, I asked my sweetheart, Isaac, if he would watch our boys while I soaked in the tub, and he obliged to my wishes.

Quickly, I darted off to the bathroom and filled the tub with very warm water and silky bubble bath. As I waited for the tub to fill, I peered into the vanity mirror and brushed my thick brown hair perfectly into place. Then I touched up my make-up by dusting rose blush onto my pale freckled Irish cheeks.

After a while of obsessing with my presentation, the tub was about full, so I slipped into it. The cleansing water warmed my long, thin body, and I felt very relaxed, without a worry in the world.

Then without thinking, I began washing my face and neck with slippery soap. Next, I ran my soapy fingers over each breast in circular motions, as I always unconsciously did during my baths, in order to feel for any unusual lumps. Suddenly, as I washed my right lower breast, I jumped. Something hurt, so I slowly palpated the breast again with my all-telling fingertips. I gasped with horror. My fingers defined a tiny very hard immobile one-quarter by one-eighth of an inch rectangular shaped lump. Panicked, my heart thumped wildly as I whispered, "Oh, my God, this must be cancer! Why couldn't I have found this lump sooner? Oh no, I must be cursed with my paternal grandmother's bad genetics. She had breast cancer in her fifties and died of a cancer recurrence in her seventies! But I'm only in my thirties and too young to die." Suddenly, my deep-set blue eyes sunk in frantic, helter-skelter fear as I anxiously yelled, "Isaac, get in here!" Seconds later, my husband's tall, husky figure flew into the bathroom, while I was still in the bathtub.

"What's wrong?" he shouted, with wide, curious brown eyes.

I gasped and pointed to the right lower breast as I cried, "I have a breast lump here. I'm scared to death. What should I do?" In the midst of my frenzy, I was hoping that my very smart husband, who had twelve years of experience as a medical doctor, would be in a position to shed some light on the mysterious lump.

"Okay, calm down, and let me feel the lump," Isaac said with concern. Then he knelt down at the bathtub and palpated the lump that I pointed out to him. "I feel the lump, but I don't know what to make of it. You'll need to see Dr. Peter Loh to assess this. He's an excellent, experienced surgeon, and I've sent him many patients with breast lumps over the years. Dr. Loh is the best doctor in town for this type of problem."

"How will Dr. Loh know if this is cancerous?" I asked anxiously in profound puzzlement, as I had never had something like a breast lump before.

"I don't assess and diagnose breast lumps. I send all my patients to Dr. Loh for that, and he'll be able to tell what this is. He takes breast lumps out all the time, and he'll know what to do, by just feeling this," Isaac said as he exited the bathroom.

In panic, I quickly jumped out of the tub, put some clothes on, and headed after Isaac. When I found him, I stared nervously at him with big, wide eyes. Finally, I managed to say, "I'm so scared and can't help but think the worst here."

"Robin, it's very common for young women, in their thirties like you, to have breast lumps, and most of these breast lumps turn out to be only benign cysts."

"Really, I didn't know that," I stated with relief, hoping I would not be one of the rare unlucky ones. So do you think this is a cyst?"

"Well, it's probably a cyst, but you need to have this checked with your gynecologist and have a mammogram," advised Isaac.

"Right, I want a mammogram as soon as possible, but it will take forever to get an appointment with my gynecologist and that will delay this mammo. Come on, Isaac, I've got to get this test as soon as possible so that I can be at peace. Can't you order the mammo right away for me?"

"I'd rather not get involved with this," said Isaac.

"Please, hon? This is very important to me."

"Well, okay," said Isaac, somewhat reluctantly. "You'll require a mammogram with ultrasound."

"Oh, thanks, I really appreciate your help, but why do I need an ultrasound?" I asked, thinking a mammogram was the diagnostic test for breast cancer determination.

"Breast ultrasound is routine with mammography for breast lump evaluation. I'll have it scheduled for you tomorrow."

"Great, hon, the sooner the better."

I was still very antsy about the lump, despite the fact that the mammogram test was to take place the very next day. Therefore, I gave my big sister a buzz on the phone, hoping she would have some sound sisterly advice or she would say something to make me feel calmer.

Unfortunately, she only suggested, in an all so serious tone, that I get the lump checked out by a doctor as soon as possible. By the time the conversation ended, I was still feeling very worried.

In fact, my mind was freaking, as if I was standing on the edge of a skyscraper, so I called my mom, hoping she would calm me down. Fortunately, she was very cool about my new breast lump, telling me that it was probably just a cyst, since it hurt. At the same time, she could not manage to hide her anxiety and asked me to call her back with an update after the mammogram.

Still feeling nervous, I called a very good young Christian friend of mine, Joye, for some encouragement and prayer. She ended up telling me that she currently had a bunch of tiny breast lumps herself that her doctor had diagnosed as being only benign cysts. Having heard that she had breast lumps that were benign, made me feel a bit calmer, but I did not know what to make of the fact that she had many lumps, but I had just one.

Worried still, I telephoned my pastor's wife for prayer. She was a little upset when she heard I had a breast lump and shouted in my ear to get a mammogram. Her anxiety aggravated my already chaotic state of mind, but I am sure she meant well.

Finally, I decided that phone calls were not helping me feel any calmer, so I tried to vent out my anxiety through work. I kept busy cleaning, cooking, and caring for my young children for the rest of the day with a detached mind.

By evening fall, I prayed with my children as usual before our bedtime, requesting God to protect me and give me a good diagnosis.

Sensitive Neo got upset when he heard my prayer request, and big tears rolled down his face. I consoled him by telling him, what I truly believed, that God would protect me.

The following morning, I woke up in a panic, thinking about my breast lump. I nervously looked for Isaac, but then remembered that he had off from work and had gone to hunt on the mountain behind our home since it was opening day of whitetail deer hunting season. In my frenzy, I somehow managed to feed my boys and get the older ones out the door for school. Then I stared out of the window and into our backyard, waiting for Isaac to return, ever so anxious for him to arrange my radiology appointment.

A long hour later, Isaac rolled his all-terrain hunting vehicle up to our back porch, arriving back very early for the first day of hunting season. Inside the back of his vehicle lay a lifeless mature doe. I cringed at the sight of the dead animal, and at the same time, I thanked God that Isaac had gotten his game. Now I did not feel so guilty about Isaac taking part of his hunting vacation time to help me with my breast problems.

After Isaac cleaned up his deer mess, he meandered into the house, looking unusually rattled. Then he grabbed the telephone with anxious, darting eyes as he set up my appointment for that very afternoon at the Cedar's Hospital Mammography Center.

Suddenly, knowing that my appointment was this near, I felt my body tense up. Full of fright, I sent anxious prayers to heaven. "God, please help me, and don't let this lump be cancerous."

Unfortunately, even my prayers failed to calm me, and I was a nervous wreck, waiting for my mammography and ultrasound tests. To help decrease my anxiety, I concentrated on looking my best for the appointment, while Isaac watched Jay. I styled my hair nicely, put on some bright make-up and got dressed in a pretty skirt and sweater. I also loaded myself with fancy jewelry, thinking that a nice appearance would signal to the medical staff to notice me and take good care of me.

Then Isaac came into the bedroom blurting, "Come on, Robin, you're taking too long to get ready. You better hurry along. I've been watching Jay this morning just so you could be on time."

"Oh, wait a minute hon, I'm almost ready. Is Jay okay?"

"Yes, don't worry about him. I'm going to watch Jay while you go to the mammography test. That way, you and the mammography medical staff can concentrate on the tests without the distraction of a toddler."

"Thanks, Isaac. That's a good idea. I hope I don't get lost looking for the mammography department, as I've never been there."

"You won't. The Cedar's Hospital Mammography Center is in the same building as my office but on the first floor instead of the third. I'm sure you'll find the department easily, and you can find parking in the lot just outside of the building."

"Okay, but I'm so nervous."

"You'll be fine. The mammography department is very nice, newly decorated, and you'll like it. I'll be praying for you, Robin."

Before I knew it, I was miraculously at the hospital mammography center, still I felt somewhat lost and bewildered. Thankfully, a nurse with gray hair who had the look of mature medical experience greeted me and guided me to an exam room. Then she instructed me to change into a patient gown and recline on the examination table. Next, she thoroughly palpated my breasts. When she found the lump, she said, "Oh yes, honey, I definitely feel that," as she placed a small black X on the lump with a felt-tip pen.

The next thing I knew, the nurse walked me into a finely decorated pink wallpapered room. Nonetheless, a chill of dread and gloom lingered in the middle of the room where a large cold metal mammogram machine hovered. The sight of it made my hands sweat, knowing I was about to get my first mammogram ever. In fear, I silently prayed to God that my mammogram would be normal and not show cancer.

Then a young female mammography technician entered the room, introduced herself, and explained that the mammogram test would be quick and painless. However, the very next instant she pulled my small A-cupped breasts so much in order to fit them in between the compression plates of the machine that I felt like my boobs were going to rip off. When the painful ordeal was finally over, the technician left me for several eternal minutes to see if the films turned out. When she finally returned, she insisted on two repeat photos of my sensitive breast with the lump, informing me that the previous pictures were not clear. More torturous testing and radiation exposure certainly did not please me. Nonetheless, I kept my mouth shut, as I was anxious to have accurate test results.

When the mammography pictures were finally finished, in trepidation, I asked the technician if I would have the test results the same day. She assured me that I would have the report following the breast ultrasound. An escort then led me to another part of the hospital for that test.

Unfortunately, once we reached the ultrasound area, another patient was occupying the test room. There was no waiting area, so my escort left me in an icy cool hallway near the exam room door. I stood there alone, for what seemed like eternity, and franticly waited for my mammogram report and ultrasound.

Finally, about twenty minutes later, the ultrasound door swung open with someone calling my name. Nervously, I darted into the room and met a female technician who seemed young and somewhat inexperienced. She had me put on a new gown and recline on the exam table. Then she rolled a warm gel-covered ultrasound transducer over my tender lump several times.

I watched the ultrasound monitor intently and with great interest, without the slightest bit of knowledge of what I was seeing. Antsy with curiosity, I asked if everything was all right. The technician said, however, that she could not comment and the doctor would speak to me soon.

A few minutes later, a busy looking physician carrying papers in his hands, briskly walked through the doorway. His long, narrow, slightly wrinkled face greeted me with a shy, reserved smile. As he approached me, I anxiously said, "Hello, doctor, was the ultrasound normal?"

Then the doctor stated, "Hi, Robin, I'm Dr. Covington. I just looked over your mammogram, and it's fine."

"Shwoo, I'm so glad to hear that. I've been so upset since I found the lump yesterday."

"Uh-huh, well, I understand your anxiety. So you're Dr. Gray's wife. I know your husband very well."

"Yes, I thought you knew my husband," I stated with relief, thinking I would get outstanding care from the doctor since I was a known entity.

Then Dr. Covington sat down and announced, "I also looked over some of the live ultrasound images of your breast lump from a monitor in an adjacent room, which look fine too. I only see a cyst. However, I want to assess the breast lump myself with the ultrasound transducer. Please point to where the lump is for me."

"It's right here in the lower right part of my breast," I nervously stated as I placed my index finger on top of the lump.

Then Dr. Covington thoroughly palpated the lump with his fingertips. "Oh yes, I feel the lump. Let's see what that looks like on the ultrasound monitor." Then he rolled the transducer back and forth over my tender breast lump with very intense pressure while he studied the ultrasound monitor.

"Ouch, easy, the lump is very sensitive!" I shouted as I squirmed in pain and nearly fell off of the exam table.

"Sorry, Robin, I must continue. I want to make sure of what I'm seeing," he stated as he continued probing with hard pressure.

"Oh no, is the lump cancerous?" I asked nervously as my heart galloped and my body shook like a leaf.

Finally, Dr. Covington stopped and calmly stated, "The ultrasound identifies only a benign cyst in your lower breast."

"Oh, I see. Then is everything all right?"

"Yes, the tests are fine, but I suggest long-term follow-up by a surgeon. That's what I normally recommend when a lump can be felt."

"Okay, I'll check this out with a surgeon, and I'm glad the tests are fine," I stated with relief.

Then Dr. Covington headed for the exit door of the exam room and stated, "I'll phone your husband with the results."

"Thanks, you may reach him at our home phone number today since he has off from work."

Once the doctor was gone, I thanked God for the good report and rushed home in my car to give Isaac the good news. When I got to my house, my husband greeted me at the kitchen door and anxiously asked me, "How did everything go at the hospital, Robin?"

"Thank God it went fine," I announced as I entered the house. "The radiologist didn't find cancer on the mammogram or ultrasound, but he did recommend long-term follow-up with a surgeon since he could feel the lump. I guess he just wants to be sure everything is okay."

"Well, I just spoke to Dr. Covington myself, and he told me the same thing," announced Isaac. "He also seemed to think that Dr. Loh would be an excellent surgeon for you to see, so I will help you arrange that appointment."

"Okay, thanks. Wow, I'm just so happy the tests are okay. I'm going to call my mother right now to let her know that the things went well today with my breast exams. Is Jay okay? Where's he anyway?"

"He's fine, go call your mother. I'll look after Jay for a bit."

I quickly dialed the long-distance phone number to Baltimore, Maryland. Then my mom answered the phone, "Hello?"

"Hi, Mom, this is Robin."

"Oh hi, Robin, how did the tests go?"

"Things look good, Mom, and the mammogram didn't find any cancer."

"Praise the Lord - thank you, Jesus."

"Yes, thank God! Mom, I can't believe now that I was so scared about the lump. How in the world could cancer fit in my small breasts anyway?" I stated jokingly.

"Well, I'm glad everything worked out well for you."

"Mom, the radiologist did recommend that I see a general surgeon for a long period of time to follow the breast lump. I guess he wants to make sure that I'm taken well care of. Isaac recommended his favorite surgeon and colleague, Dr. Loh. Isaac says he's a great doctor and knows his stuff. Also, Isaac knows Dr. Loh personally and used to hunt woodchucks on his land. So I'm sure the good doctor will look out for me. "

"Oh, I'm so glad that you have someone you can trust to look at the lump. I'll be praying for you, honey."

"Well, thanks, Mom. I appreciate it, and I will call you back."

When I got off the phone, Isaac said, "What did your mother say?"

"Well, she was relieved, just like me. Anyway, if my radiology tests are fine, what exactly can Dr. Loh tell me that the tests haven't already revealed? I don't get why I have to see him."

"A surgeon is the final authority and expert in the assessment of breast lumps," informed Isaac. "I'm going to call Dr. Loh's office right now to make sure you have that surgical appointment as soon as possible."

"Thanks, Isaac. I'll feel better once he, too, has verified that everything is fine."

Unfortunately, the soonest appointment turned out to be two days later. The long two-day wait caused a build-up of anxiety so by the morning of the appointment, I was very jumpy. At least Isaac was off from work and home to support me, that day. He not only reassured me that everything would be okay, but he volunteered to watch little Jay at home, so I could listen attentively during my doctor's appointment without the fuss of a two-year-old.

When I finally got to the surgeon's office, a friendly secretary greeted me and handed me a history form to fill out. I found the last seat in a crowded little waiting room with the odd thought that the crowd was the sign of a good doctor awaiting us. Full of anxiety, my sweaty fingers went to work, scribbling out answers to the medical questionnaire form. Date- Nov. 20, 2000; Age- 38; Weight- thin, 129 lb.; Height- 5'7''; Current Patient Medical History- none; Use of

Alcohol or Drugs- none; Use of Tobacco- none; Breast Problems- Right lower quadrant hard breast lump...

About fifteen minutes into my wait, a friendly middle-aged female nurse introduced herself as Molly. Then she walked me to a small, neat exam room, and I noticed her nametag had R.N. on it. Therefore, I mentioned that I was a registered nurse, too, but I had not worked in nearly ten years. She commented that she was nearly done with her nurse-practitioner postgraduate studies, and consequently, I was impressed and more at ease, with the knowledge that I was in the hands of a well- educated healthcare professional.

Molly seated me in the exam room, and I explained my breast lump concerns to her. She seemed attentive but not alarmed about the lump as she jotted down a few notes for Dr. Loh. When she was through with my patient history, she announced in a sweet voice that she would be back soon with Dr. Loh.

Meanwhile, I changed into the patient gown and waited like a frozen popsicle in anticipation of the doctor's opinion. A few moments later, Dr. Loh entered the room. I looked up to him with great respect and noticed the look of experience that Isaac had mentioned. He had a very thick head of short winter-white hair and pale, wrinkled skin that creased deeply around his eyes and mouth deeply as he smiled. His perfectly tailored white lab coat fit snuggly around him to accentuate his older but fit, tall frame. He spoke with mature confidence and stated, "Hello, Robin, it's been a while since I've seen you. How are you? The last time I saw you was years ago when you were working at the hospital. I see here on your notes that you're here due to a breast lump."

"Hi, Dr. Loh, it's good to see you again. Yes, I'm concerned about a breast lump that I found just three days ago, in my right, lower, outer breast. The lump frightened me so much that Isaac ordered an immediate mammogram/ultrasound of my breasts. According to the radiologist, Dr. Covington, who I saw two days ago, the mammogram and ultrasound were normal, but he recommended long-term follow-up with a surgeon to be sure everything is fine. So, Isaac highly recommended you."

"Uh-huh," smiled Dr. Loh. "Since you found the lump three days ago, has it changed size?"

"Since the mammogram and ultrasound, which may have flared things up, the breast lump seems slightly smaller. Even so, I'm nervous because my paternal grandmother died of breast cancer."

"Well, Robin, the fact that your grandmother had breast cancer is not significant because only first-degree relatives, such as one's siblings or mother, increase the risk for breast cancer; not second-degree relatives such as grandmothers."

"Well, I'm glad to hear that."

"Let's see what's going on here. Please lie down flat on the exam table," instructed Dr. Loh. Then he stepped up to the table and thoroughly palpated my right breast with his fingertips. Then he calmly stated, "I feel the breast lump in the right lower breast, here."

"Yes, that's a bit tender, Dr. Loh," I said as I wondered what lay ahead, hoping everything would be fine.

The doctor continued his examination by palpating my left and right breast, along with the axillary lymph nodes under both armpits. Finally, when he was done, he calmly stated, "I didn't find anything suspicious, and there are no masses under your armpit, which is good. Nonetheless, I'll check the right breast with the ultrasound."

"Another ultrasound?" I asked in surprise since I had just had the test and wondering why another would be required.

"Yes, I want to be certain that everything is fine. I'll be back in a moment with the machine." A few minutes later, Dr. Loh was back, wheeling in the portable ultrasound monitor. He parked it behind my exam table, out of my sight, and plugged it in. Then he ran the ultrasound transducer over my breast lump several times, as he stared at the ultrasound monitor very quietly and seriously.

All the while, Dr. Loh's silent probing made me very anxious. I wanted to ask him if everything was okay, but I did not want to interrupt his concentration. Therefore, I studied his face intently to see if concern was written on it. However, it was an old poker face and gave no clues.

Finally, Dr. Loh announced, "Your breast lump appears cystic, and I don't see anything suspicious."

"I'm so glad to hear that," I blurted, as I stared into Dr. Loh's steely, blue-gray eyes that hid behind distorting spectacles. "Dr. Loh, I have some small amounts of brown nipple discharge from just my right breast, the same breast with the lump, that I'm concerned about. Is this normal with cystic breasts?" I inquired.

Dr. Loh bobbed his head up and down like a yoyo with assurance. "A lot of young women have nipple drainage in childbearing years, and it's normal and nothing to worry about."

"Good, I'm relieved to hear that."

Then Dr. Loh walked to the end of my exam table while I was still reclined flat out on the exam table. I looked straight up to him with great respect and expectation as he announced, "After examining your breasts, nothing is suspicious by physical exam or breast ultrasound. The lump appears cystic, and this is what we call f i b r o - c y - s t i c breast condition, which requires no medical treatment."

"Good," I said with relief. I had never heard of 'fibrocystic breast condition.' However, by the sound of it, it was a fancy word for a benign cystic breast.

Dr. Loh continued, "Fibrocystic breast condition is a harmless condition. In fact, it's very common in young women, of your age, with fluctuating hormones. You can reduce the caffeine in your diet, which may elevate or reduce the cystic condition."

"Well, I certainly would like to get rid of this, so I'll eliminate the caffeine in my diet. I'm not a huge coffee drinker, but unfortunately, I have been drinking more than usual, lately."

"Uh-huh, well certainly a cup of coffee a day would be permissible, but please do not drink too much. I'd like to have some follow-up of the lump in about three weeks from now. From now to the next appointment, you'll find that your lump may gradually change in size, due to normal menstrual hormonal fluctuations. However, call my office sooner for an appointment if the lump suddenly explodes in size.

Well, I'll be seeing you in three weeks, and have a wonderful Thanksgiving tomorrow."

"I certainly will, and thank you so much for your help, doctor. You have a great holiday too."

With disarmed fears, I joyfully went home and informed Isaac about the benign diagnosis. He was glad and told me that Dr. Loh had just phoned him with the fibrocystic diagnosis as well. Overwhelmed with joy and feeling blessed, we thanked God.

Then I ecstatically called my mother and informed her of the fibrocystic diagnosis. Of course, she, too, was elated about the benign findings.

After I got off the phone, Isaac got out his medical text titled Harrison's Principles of Internal Medicine and read about fibrocystic breast disease. He shared with me that my breast lump fit the fibrocystic description, which only further assured me of Dr. Loh's diagnosis.

The next day was Thanksgiving Day, and I was exhausted from having had a hectic week with seeing various doctors. Therefore, I decided not to have my in-laws at my home for the holidays, as I usually did. However, our own small family of five celebrated with joy over my benign diagnosis.

The following week, Isaac informed me that he had received a medical consult note on me from Dr. Loh, which documented my visit and the fibrocystic breast diagnosis. Of course, the note to my husband, the verbal fibrocystic diagnosis to me, and Dr. Loh's reassuring phone call to my husband fully assured me of a benign diagnosis.

Nonetheless, I was anxious to get rid of my lump, so I began working very hard at eliminating almost all caffeine from my diet, except for an occasional Hershey's Milk Chocolate Kiss, which was one of my favorite candies. I missed my daily morning coffee and evening hot cocoa; however, I was determined to eliminate caffeine, as recommended by Dr. Loh.

My husband also tried to help me with getting rid of my breast lump. He gave me a letter from the Lauren Breast Clinic that one of his patients had given to him concerning the treatment for her fibrocystic breast condition. Isaac suggested that I could try it, and share the recommendations with Dr. Loh at the follow-up visit.

When I read the note, I found that a daily regimen of one vitamin E tablet and one evening primrose oil tablet sometimes eliminates breast cysts. Anxious to resolve my cyst, I obtained the over-the-counter supplements and immediately started the regimen.

A few days after taking the supplements, I glanced at the letter again to make sure that I was correctly following the regimen. It was at that moment when I first noticed the phone number of the out-of-town breast clinic, which was printed written in the letterhead of the note. Suddenly, I thought it would be a good idea to call the clinic and see what they had to offer for surgical breast assessment. Therefore, I dialed the long-distance number. An operator answered, "Hello this is the breast clinic."

"Hi, my name is Robin Gray. My husband is a medical internist and practices a few hours from your facility. I've been diagnosed with fibrocystic condition by a local surgeon, and I was wondering if you have any surgeons at your clinic to evaluate my breast lump for a second opinion?"

"No, we don't employ surgeons. We only have radiologists that work here. Perhaps one of them can look at your breast lump. Would you like to schedule an appointment?"

"Well, I've already seen a radiologist, and he couldn't treat me further since my mammogram was fine. He indicated that I needed long-term surgical care for my palpable lump. Consequently, I'm looking for a breast surgeon, not a radiologist. Are you sure you don't have a breast surgeon that could look at the lump?"

"No ma'am, --only radiologists are employed here."

"Oh I see," I commented, thinking it was odd that a breast clinic wouldn't employ a breast surgeon. "Could you or a nurse please give me the name of any surgical breast expert in your area who you make referrals to?"

"No ma'am, that's against our policy. You got to get the referral from your doctor."

"Oh, can you drop me the name of someone who is an experienced breast surgeon? You don't need to make the referral for me."

"Sorry, we can't give out names."

I hung up the phone feeling discouraged, and I thought the clinic was not very helpful with their put-off and impersonal attitude. Consequently, I felt very lucky to have Dr. Loh, as my local surgeon, who, according to Isaac, was an outstanding doctor with years of experience in breast assessment. Furthermore, I felt assured that my husband's colleague would certainly offer me the best medical care possible.

Unfortunately, unknown to me, I was beginning to be led down a perverse path of medical errors. Early diagnosis and treatment of the malignant growth within me was beginning to slip through my fingers, the same fingers that had found the breast lump in the first place. Sadly, I was becoming one of thousands of young women in the United States that suffer a physician-related delayed diagnosis of breast cancer. (1)

Chapter Learning Tips

To those who have breast lumps, take a deep breath and realize that many lumps turn out to be benign. At the same time, breast cancer misdiagnosis is common in women, especially those that are forty-five years old and younger. All women should carefully have their breast lumps assessed. The following list may help you cope and find the right diagnosis.

1. Discovery of a breast lump can be traumatic. Obtain the support of friends and family, and try to get someone with another set of ears to go with you to your doctor appointment(s).

2. You are already ahead in the game of avoiding a breast misdiagnosis as you know that breast cancer misdiagnosis is a possible risk, especially for younger women.

3. Consider anti-anxiety medication if you are too overwhelmed while trying to determine if your breast lump is cancerous.

4. Consider holding off on caffeine products and any estrogen medications, which may aggravate breast lumps.

5. Do not let a misdiagnosis slip through your fingers. See my postscript guide for steps to avoid a breast misdiagnosis. By taking time to educate yourself with my guide you may feel more calm and in control of your health.

Chapter 2

Doctors' Deceptive Web

The leading cause of physician delay in diagnosis of breast cancer continues to be inappropriate reassurance that a mass is benign without biopsy, with or without reliance on mammography.

_Archives of Internal Medicine, June 24, 2002

December of 2000 rang in, bringing with it a foggy ominous mass. Snows followed the mass about, dumping a thick whitewash covering all over the valley where I lived. The downpour of snow around my home was so thick that distant vision was impossible; it would have taken a knife to see through it.

However, my family and I hardly noticed the bad weather. We were enjoying the holiday season by decorating the tree, sending out Christmas cards, and doing a ton of holiday baking. In between those activities, I rushed about doing holiday shopping and gift-wrapping until I almost dropped.

During the busy season, I had no worries about my breast lump since Dr. Loh told me that it was only fibrocystic condition. However, I did check the size of my breast lump during my daily baths and only found that it did not change much in size except it seemed a tiny bit bigger during my period.

Therefore, when I finally arrived at Dr. Loh's office for my three-week follow-up in early December, I was calm, thinking my lump was fine. In fact, as I waited to see the doctor, I peacefully watched a cartoon television series, Bob the Builder, with my young son, Jay, by my side.

After about twenty-five minutes of waiting, the nurse, Molly, shouted my name out. Then she led us back to an exam room where I informed her that my breast lump was about same size. Molly smiled, as she made some medical chart notations. Then she left me with a patient gown to place on and departed for Dr. Loh.

Minutes later the much-respected doctor finally entered the room. He sternly nodded at Jay, who was quietly playing with his fire truck. Then he turned to me with a warmer glow and stated, "Hello, how's everything going?"

"Okay, but I am still concerned about my breast lump. It may have been a bit bigger during my period, but now it seems nearly the same size as when I last saw you."

Dr. Loh nodded and assured, "Well, that's fibrocystic breast condition. It can fluctuate in size with the menstrual cycle, as yours has."

"Oh, okay, but I still have a small amount of nipple drainage from the right breast…"

Quickly, before I could finish, Dr. Loh interrupted, "Yes, that's normal. A lot of young women in child bearing years have nipple drainage."

"Uh-huh, that's what I thought you said in the previous visit," I quickly blurted, as I felt somewhat embarrassed for bringing up the same question twice.

"Well, let me just take a look at the lump today," announced Dr. Loh as he and his nurse approached me, and I laid out flat on the exam table. Then the doctor palpated my breasts, the right breast lump, and my axillary lymph node. Finally, after his seemly thorough physical breast assessment, I quickly covered myself up with the gown and asked, "Is everything okay?"

Then Dr. Loh looked me straight in the eye and announced, "Oh yes, this feels the same. This is fibrocystic breast condition, and I don't see anything that is suspicious."

"Well, I'm glad that everything is fine, Dr. Loh," I replied as I sat up from the exam table. "Isaac gave me some literature about fibrocystic breast condition from the Lauren Breast Clinic located out-of-town further north. I have been taking their recommended regimen of vitamin E and evening primrose oil to help resolve the cyst. What do you think? Will it help?"

"Well, I've heard of these regimens being recommended by the Lauren Breast Clinic. You can try it, but it really doesn't have any proven effectiveness," he stated with a dubious smile.

"Oh, I see, then perhaps I should stop taking them," I muttered, feeling somewhat awkward that I had taken the unendorsed supplements.

Dr. Loh smiled and asked, "Any more questions or concerns?"

"Well, I do want to tell you that I called the Lauren Breast Clinic, after seeing their letter on the treatment of fibrocystic breast condition. I wanted to see if they had a surgeon to render a second opinion on my breast lump. However, they told me that they had radiologists, not surgeons; therefore, they couldn't make any kind of surgical appointment for me. But I assume you are comfortable and able to assess the lump. Right?"

"Oh, yes," Dr. Loh assured with a wide smile and nod. "I can take care of this for you. Fibrocystic breast condition is a well-known and common condition that I'm familiar with."

"Good," I said with a smile as I was glad of the doctor's assurances.

"Is there anything else today that I can help you with?" asked Dr. Loh.

"Should I still limit the caffeine? I have been trying to reduce my caffeine, as you instructed, but I don't know if it's helping since I still have the cyst."

"I would suggest that you continue caffeine limitation, which is the recommended for fibrocystic condition. It may or may not help, but stick with it."

"Sure."

"Good. Since things are fine today, and this continues to be fibrocystic condition, I will not need to see you again until a three-month follow-up appointment."

"Thanks, I'll see you then."

When I got home, I called Isaac at his office. Of course, he had already heard from Dr. Loh and was happy with the continued benign diagnosis. I was glad that Dr. Loh had discussed the visit with Isaac, confirming that the lump was fine.

As January coldly blew into my life, I nearly forgot about my benign lump. I was very busy with many activities revolving around my kids. In the evenings, I was busy taking the older boys to ice-skating lessons and assisting them with homework. During the days, I taught Jay the Abeka Pre-Kindergarten Home Schooling Program, and I often took him to the public library to pick up pre-school reading books. I even remember picking up a few Albert Einstein and Thomas Edison books for the older boys, too, in order to encourage them academically. Ironically, I missed the section of the library that contained breast cancer books, believing my erroneous benign diagnosis.

The weeks mounted on in January and February, I continued to check and palpate my breast lump every few weeks, monitoring its size. During these checks, the lump was about the same as my prior visit, so I thought my breast was fine.

Then when March arrived, I noticed that my breast lump felt a little bit bigger than usual. I did not panic though, thinking it was fluctuating a bit in size with my caffeine intake or hormones as Dr. Loh said it would.

Then on the morning of my follow-up appointment, which was on March 12, 2001, I noticed that my breast lump felt even larger, nearly double from its previous size in November 2000. Somewhat disturbed by the enlargement, I read about fibrocystic breast condition in some of Isaac's medical books, Harrison's Medicine and The Merck Manual, just before I left for Dr. Loh's office. Unfortunately, the books did not discuss whether cysts could enlarge or not, which worried me more.

When I got to Dr. Loh's office, I told the nurse, Molly, that I was worried about my breast lump and that it seemed consistently bigger. She did not say much though, only making a few notations in my medical chart, and left for Dr. Loh.

After a bit of a wait, Dr. Loh entered the exam room with a big smile and stated, "Hello, it's been a few months." Then he looked at Jay, who was in the corner of the room dressed in tiny bib overalls and drawing on his magic coloring board. Full of smiles, Dr. Loh asked my son, "Are you working hard on your writing? Are you trying to be smart, huh?" In response, Jay stared silently at the strange doctor.

I nervously said, "Dr. Loh, my breast lump might fluctuate in size during my periods, but it also has gotten bigger and I'm concerned. Is this usual with fibrocystic breasts?"

"Yes, fibrocystic lumps can harmlessly get bigger in size due to the female hormones. Let's see what the lump feels like." Then he had me lay flat out on the exam table and palpated my breasts, the lump, and axillary lymph nodes. When he finished, he smiled while he announced, "This is still only benign fibrocystic condition."

"Good, I'm glad to hear that, but are you sure it's safe that the lump is bigger?" I asked with concern.

"Well, in fibrocystic breast condition, lumps can get quite large, five centimeters or more, and still be harmless."

"Oh, I didn't know that. Will the lump ever regress or disappear at some point?" I asked inquisitively.

"Fibrocystic lumps may enlarge without concern during the years of menstruation and usually, but not always, disappear once menopause begins," assured Dr. Loh.

"Uh-huh. Well, could my fibrocystic lump ever, at anytime, increase my chances of breast cancer developing?"

With a confident tone and a reassuring smile, Dr. Loh said, "Fibrocystic lumps do not increase one's risk for breast cancer."

"Good. Then you are sure that everything is okay?"

"Yes, this is fibrocystic condition, and I don't see anything suspicious. However, due to the slight lump enlargement, I'll do a fine needle aspiration."

"Oh my," I said with surprise. I had never heard of a fine needle aspiration or seen one done. Therefore, I was worried about what was to come next. However, before I could think further, Dr. Loh quickly opened a needle and syringe and plunged it piercingly into my breast lump, as he steadied his fingers on my right lower breast. Then Dr. Loh pulled back on the syringe to aspirate and vacuum the lump's contents, and I jerked my leg in response to the pain, wondering why the doctor did not use numbing medication. Dr. Loh then inserted another needle slightly higher, aspirating it in the same painful fashion.

"Ah, that hurts!" I yelled.

Suddenly, Jay darted up to the exam table, opposite Dr. Loh. His tiny head barely bobbed over the table, as his big blue prophetic eyes looked up at Dr. Loh and announced, "Don't hurt my mama!"

"Jay, I'll be okay. The doctor is almost done here, and he's placing some nice Band-Aids on me. Go back in your chair and draw." However,

Jay continued to stay by my side and tightly held onto my leg, as he stared Dr. Loh down.

Meanwhile, I wondered if I should look at the syringe, full of fear of what I might see. However, I finally mustered up some nerve and got a quick glance of it in Dr. Loh's hand before he handed it to the nurse. Surprisingly, I noticed it contained a small amount of dark brown-green fluid. Therefore, I nervously stated, "Dr. Loh, I see that the syringe had greenish fluid in it!"

"Yes, that's fine. The green fluid is reflective of cystic condition and is a normal finding seen in fibrocystic breast condition," assured Dr. Loh with a smile.

"Oh, okay, but are you sure that the hard rectangular lump in my breast has been properly assessed?" I inquired with great concern, as I winced over my painful pierced breast.

With serious eyes, Dr. Loh assured me, "Oh yes, the fluid I aspirated from your breast is reflective of that area."

"Are you sure?" I asked intently.

Again, Dr. Loh nodded, smiled, and assured, "The fine needle aspiration has adequately assessed all areas of concern in your breast."

"You are sure?"

"Yes, I am," he insisted with a wide confident smile. "Everything has gone well today. Nothing is suspicious for cancer and you continue with fibrocystic breast condition, so I will not need to see you until six months from now for a follow-up visit."

"Well, I'm so glad everything is fine, and I'll see you in six months," I announced still in pain from the procedure. After the doctor left, I very slowly got dressed due to my sore right breast and carefully departed.

Unfortunately, as I drove home from the doctor's office, I was very uncomfortable from the bee-stinging pain of the fine needle aspiration. In fact, I had a hard time driving, and I used my right hand to put pain-relieving counter-pressure on my right pierced breast, leaving me only one free hand for driving.

When I finally got home, I immediately took some Tylenol and placed a warm soothing washcloth over the needled areas that were already forming two dime-sized blue bruises. To ease my pain further, I rested on the living-room sofa.

After a while, I telephoned my mother for a little sympathy. However, when I told my mom about my painful fine needle aspiration, she was not concerned about my pain, but she seemed frightened that I had received a fine needle aspiration. Immediately, I assured her that Dr. Loh continued with his benign fibrocystic diagnosis, even after the procedure, which eased her mind.

Once I got off the phone, my mother's initial reaction over the fine needle aspiration bothered me, and it prompted me to think about the procedure that Dr. Loh had just performed on me. Suddenly, once again, I wondered if the fine needle aspiration that Dr. Loh performed on me truly assessed my entire breast lump as he had assured. Therefore, I poked around on Isaac's medical bookshelf for a text that discussed fine needle aspiration and its assessment accuracy, but I did not find a book that explained the procedure thoroughly.

Consequently, by the time Isaac got home from work, I anxiously approached him at the doorway and asked, "Isaac, did you know I had an aspiration today on my breast lump?"

"Yes, Dr. Loh called me and said that your breast lump was only fibrocystic and nothing to worry about."

Then I followed Isaac to his bedroom and said, "I know Dr. Loh said my breast lump is not suspicious for cancer and is fibrocystic, but I'm very concerned. I just don't know if Dr. Loh truly sampled the entire lump with the fine needle aspiration procedure. When I asked Dr. Loh if he had adequately assessed my entire breast lump, he assured me that he had and said that I continued with fibrocystic breast condition. I was trying to read some of your gynecology medical books today to see if, in fact, he had done the fine needle aspiration properly and check the procedure's assessment accuracy. "

"What are you doing looking through my old out-of-date medical books for information about breast fine needle aspiration?" asked Isaac. "You can't learn proper breast assessment with just a text book. You need clinical breast experience to do that. Dr. Loh is an experienced clinical expert and has the skills for proper breast assessment. He knows what he is doing."

"Are you sure?" I wined inquisitively.

"Yes, of course, Robin," Isaac stated with serious assurance. "Dr. Loh is a stellar surgeon and handles my breast cases all the time. I've never had a problem with him. I'm just glad you have him, and I think you can trust him. Now stop worrying, he told you and me repeatedly that your breast lump is not suspicious for cancer and is only a cyst. "

When Isaac was through with his praises about Dr. Loh, I not only felt relieved and assured about the surgeon's fine needle aspiration and assessments, but I felt humbled like an all-believing child. I certainly thought my bright, compulsive physician husband would never back Dr. Loh unless he was certain about the surgeon's skills. Completely sold on Dr. Loh, I trusted my surgeon's assessments, procedures, and unequivocal benign fibrocystic diagnosis of my breast lump.

Consequently, I went about my life without anxiety about my breast lump. In fact, I took a peaceful trip in mid-April, during Easter break, back to my hometown in Baltimore, Maryland, to visit family without a thought of my benign fibrocystic lump.

The next time I remember thinking of my breast lump was in May of 2001 when I had my routine gynecology appointment with a nurse practitioner. However, even at this point, I did not worry about the lump. In fact, I informed the nurse practitioner that Dr. Loh had examined my breast lump several times and had repeatedly diagnosed it as fibrocystic breast condition and not suspicious for cancer. Furthermore, I added that I had recently had a normal mammogram, several normal ultrasounds, and a very recent fine needle aspiration by Dr. Loh, in which he continued to assure me that my breast lump was benign fibrocystic condition. The nurse practitioner seemed very satisfied with Dr. Loh assessing and following my fibrocystic breast lump and did not suggest or recommend any other referrals for my lump.

As summer approached, I did not think about my breast lump much, except during monthly self-breast exams. Even then, I did not worry about the lump, which was unchanged in size, because I trusted it was benign fibrocystic condition as Dr. Loh had told me. Like a mindless fool, I enjoyed the summer with my children without a care. We peacefully went fishing at our pond, hiking in our woods, and vacationing once again in Baltimore, Maryland, to see my family.

Then in August 2001, without warning, my mother called and informed me that my eighty-eight-year-old maternal grandmother had an aggressive cancerous breast lump that was excoriating through her skin. Immediately, I thought of my own lump, and I thanked God that it was only benign and nothing like my grandmother's lump. At the same time, I felt horrible for my grandmother. I was especially upset when I learned that she had found her breast lump nearly two years earlier, and she had chosen to keep it a secret from her family and not treat it.

Somehow, I thought that my grandmother had a fighting chance, despite her neglected lump. However, as the days passed, I learned that her cancer had spread to her lungs, causing her condition to deteriorate very quickly. Then before I knew it, she was in hospice care, and she passed on before I could even make it down to Baltimore to see her.

The death of my grandmother from the hideous thief, breast cancer, haunted me, as I thought about my own breast lump. To make matters worse, after my grandmother's death, my lump started to feel larger, almost twice as big in size from the previous visit with Dr. Loh. I told Isaac how concerned I was about my enlarging breast lump coupled with my grandmother's recent death. I also asked him if I should immediately see Dr. Loh for the lump. However, Isaac reminded me that Dr. Loh said the lump was only benign fibrocystic condition that could get larger without harm, which calmed me down. Then Isaac reassuringly added that my appointment was only several days off, and I could discuss my concerns with Dr. Loh soon. I figured Isaac was right, so I calmed down and thought it was safe to wait for my appointment.

However, by the time I ended up at Dr. Loh's office for my follow-up visit, about a week later, I was very jittery with fear. As the doctor entered the exam room, I nervously said, "Hi, Dr. Loh, I'm very anxious about my breast lump. It is definitely much bigger at about one inch by one and a half inches. I'm especially concerned since my other grandmother just died of breast cancer."

"Your grandmothers' breast cancer histories do NOT increase your risk of getting breast cancer Only first-degree relatives like sisters or mothers increase one's risk of breast cancer. Let me take a look at the lump and see what's going on," Dr. Loh announced calmly with a smile.

Then as I reclined flat on the exam table with fright, Dr. Loh palpated my breast lump, both of my breasts, and my axillary lymph nodes. Finally, he said, "I don't feel anything suspicious. I'll do another ultrasound today to be sure everything is fine."

Dr. Loh quickly exited the room and came back pushing a large ultrasound machine, which he parked behind my head. Then he rolled the ultrasound's gel-covered transducer over my breast lump several times, as he looked calmly at the monitor. Finally, he announced, "Everything on the ultrasound monitor looks fine and nothing is suspicious for cancer. This continues to be fibrocystic breast condition, which requires no treatment."

"Then everything is okay, even though the lump is larger?" I asked nervously.

"Yes, everything looks fine, and I don't identify anything suspicious for cancer. This continues to be fibrocystic breast condition. You do not require any further follow-up exams since this has been followed safely for a very long length of time. The only thing I suggest is that you obtain a mammogram a year from now, and you may contact me if any questions or problems arise."

"I'm so glad everything is okay. Thank you so much for your help."

"Certainly, it's been a pleasure. Say hi to Isaac for me."

When I got home, I excitedly called Isaac to tell him the good news; however, he had already heard from Dr. Loh with the continued benign fibrocystic diagnosis. Therefore, he was happy and told me that he knew everything would turn out fine.

When Isaac and I went to bed that night, I chatted about my visit with Dr. Loh. I shook my head and said, "Can you believe I was so upset for nothing, Isaac? I thought an enlarging lump that big would be a bad thing. That just goes to show you what little I know. Thank God, I have the expert, Dr. Loh, who knows how to assess and diagnose breast lumps and knows my lump is only benign."

"Yep, Robin, I'm certainly glad everything is fine." Then Isaac kissed me, and we joyfully celebrated the evening in romance, like a couple of newlyweds.

Unfortunately, like a brainwashed fool, I trusted Dr. Loh's assessments. My instincts were dead by faith in my doctors, and I was stuck in an invisible web of medical mistakes.

As autumn rolled in, my fall days were devoid of breast worries, while I was busy caring for my children. I was home schooling Jay, who was now three years old. In addition, during the evenings, I kept busy helping my older boys with homework, piano lessons, and evening practices for a church play.

Before I knew it, December had come, and I was busy preparing for Christmas. In the midst of the holiday rush, I did my monthly self-breast exam and my breast lump seemed slightly larger. However, I thought it was nothing to worry about since Dr. Loh had confirmed on several physician visits that it was benign fibrocystic condition and could get larger without harm. Ironically, I enjoyed the holidays with ignorant content, as my fibrocystic breast lump, whose real name was ductal carcinoma in situ, a precancerous growth, was beginning to get restless and yearned to express itself as an aggressive and potentially deadly invasive carcinoma.

Chapter Learning Tips

The surgical follow-up appointment that shortly follows your initial appointment for a breast lump is very important, especially if your lump is persistent! You must be certain that your surgeon is doing everything possible to adequately rule out any chance of cancer early-on. I believe that the following list of suggestions may help you get through the early follow-up appointment(s).

1. Have a friend or family member with you for support during the follow-up appointment(s).

2. Do not allow your first follow-up appointment to be delayed, as early diagnosis is essential. I believe you should see your physician for follow-up as soon as your diagnostic testing is completed in order to discuss the test results.

3. Discuss your fears openly about cancer with your doctor, concerns about a misdiagnosis, and need to have early diagnosis.

4. Realize that the cause of a breast misdiagnosis can be a series of assuring wrong doctor opinions from one or several doctors.

5. See my postscript guide for steps to help avoid a breast misdiagnosis.

Chapter 3

Unapologetic Delayed Diagnosis

Most victims of malpractice are given phony explanations, attributing the problem to unnamed complications, or "God's will", or a host of mysterious and inexplicable phenomena. With rare exceptions, they are never told the truth.

_Lethal Medicine, 1993

O n the mountain at my home, it was a dead dark winter in the new year of 2002. The sun hid itself from the thousands of young tree skeletons on the mountain at our home, which were smothered by layers of heavy icy snow. Under the pressure of it all, many tree limbs snapped loudly, fell and tumbled to the valley below. Piles of fallen broken pieces and ugly carnage collected on top of our ice-covered pond, failing to break through or awaken old bass, which slept and blindly lied in the deep murky pit.

My kids and I hated this harsh ugly season so we often stayed inside our home, sheltering ourselves from winter's harsh blow. Old man winter was hard to take and would have been harder without my boys. However, my kids kept my spirits bright and my mind busy. During the day, I taught Jay three-year-old pre-kindergarten studies. Then once Luke and Neo were home from school, I assisted them on their piano assignments, and the house was filled with beautiful classical melodies.

All during January and February, I was so busy with my children and enjoying life that I hardly thought about my breast lump. The rare times I did think about it was during monthly self-breast exams. However, even then, I did not dwell on my fibrocystic breast condition since it was benign and nearly the same in size from my prior doctor's visit.

Then when late March 2002 arrived, I was bathing and somewhat alarmingly noticed that my breast lump was suddenly bigger than September 2001, when I last saw Dr Loh. It was now about two inches by two inches big. Even so, I thought the enlarging mass was fine, remembering how Dr. Loh told me that fibrocystic breast condition could enlarge without harm. Although, I did make a mental note to check my enlarged breast lump again soon to see if it would regress in size after my period, which I concurrently had.

About a week later, in early April, I palpated my breast lump once again, during bath time. I was utterly shocked when I noticed that the lump was yet again larger by about another half-inch. In disbelief, I quickly stretched my fingers from one end of the lump to the other to double-check the measure of its span. Again, I was stunned, as it seemed about two and a half to three inches long! Astounded with the size of the mass, I jumped out of the tub, ran up to the bathroom mirror, and visually inspected my right breast.

Immediately, spring's sunlight gleamed from our bathroom window and shined on me brightly, illuminating my right breast, which

I thought looked maybe slightly smaller around the base, as if its defining bottom perimeter had moved ever so slightly up by a few millimeters, but I wasn't absolutely sure. As I reflected on my breast, the distant voice of my nursing professor, from many years past, returned to me. In a moment, my mind was seated in her classroom of years earlier, "Ladies and Gentlemen, sometimes pitting in a breast may be a sign of cancer; albeit, it is not your job as a nurse to diagnose." Suddenly, I felt concerned, my breast did not have any pitting, but I wondered why it seemed maybe slightly smaller at the base. I may have worried more, but I remembered that Dr. Loh had ascertained a benign fibrocystic diagnosis for the lump several times. Still, I wanted to speak to Isaac about my enlarged lump, but he was at work, so I paced the house nervously with little Jay by my side.

When my husband finally got home, I followed him to our bedroom like a frightened little dog. Then as he was changing out of his fancy work clothes, I blurted, "Isaac I have some questions about my breast lump. I know Dr. Loh said it could get larger, but it seems huge now. Can you please feel my breast lump?" I stripped off my shirt and bra and pointed out the borders of the lump. Then Isaac felt it.

"That lump seems to be a lot bigger. You've got to call Dr. Loh back to have him check it out."

"Why do you think it's so much bigger? Is everything okay? Have you ever had a patient with a benign lump this big?" I demanded.

"I don't know why that thing feels so much bigger. You better go see Dr. Loh, the expert."

"Oh no," I wined; "now you've got me worried."

"Well, Dr. Loh did say your lump was only fibrocystic and could get larger without harm. Just get it checked out, and we'll feel better about it, Robin."

"Right, I'll feel better after he sees it again. I just hope this is still fibrocystic!"

The next morning, still very upset, I called Dr. Loh's office about the enlarged lump and got a follow-up appointment, which was just a few days off. Unfortunately, when that appointment arrived, Jay and I were ill with a vomiting virus, and I had to postpone the appointment for a few more days.

In the meantime, I grew very anxious over the recent lump enlargement. I called my mother for a little support; however, I was never able to share my concerns with her, as she was still grieving from her mother's death. Of course, my mother's grief over her mother's breast cancer death only made me feel worse.

In fact, my mind was so worried over my breast lump, my grandmothers' breast cancers, and my mother's grief that I could hardly relax or sleep. Isaac tried to calm me, stating that Dr. Loh said the lump was only benign, but I was still upset.

When Jay and I finally made it to my appointment with Dr. Loh on, April 18, 2002, I felt like a zombie due to the prior insomnia. In fact, I was almost too tired to reflect on my fears concerning my much-enlarged lump, as I waited in the exam room to be seen by Dr. Loh. When he finally entered the room, he looked calm, sophisticated, and full of self-assurance, whereas I felt weary and worn. Then the bright doctor asked, "How are you?"

"Not too good. I'm very upset about my breast lump, which has recently gotten much bigger. I asked Isaac why it was so much bigger, but he said he didn't know and that I had to see you. Can you believe I'm married to a doctor, and he can't give me a clue as to why this is so much bigger?" I stated half jokingly, shaking my head back and forth in disbelief.

"Oh, yes, that's because you are the wife. I'm the same way with my wife," assured Dr. Loh. "Even though we are doctors, we can't really be objective with our spouses, offering medical diagnoses or opinions."

"Right, that's why I'm here to see you."

"Well, let's see what's going on with your lump. Please recline on the exam table," announced Dr. Loh.

Suddenly Dr. Loh and his nurse approached me. I stated nervously, "I'm so upset over the large size of my breast lump. When I was in fifth grade, a boy grabbed my right breast with pliers and gave me a breast bruising injury. Could this be the reason the lump is so big now? Also, when I breastfeed, lactation was slower on the right side. I always thought it was sluggish because my breast was smaller on the right side, and it was harder to get the baby to latch on and nurse. However, perhaps something else was going on. I don't know what's going on, but I'm really upset about my enlarged breast lump."

"Well, it sounds like you had some mean boy in your fifth grade class and nothing to worry about now," Dr. Loh assured with a smile. Then he began palpating my breast lump, breasts, and armpit areas. When he was done, he announced, "This feels the same-fibrocystic.

However, due to your concerns and the enlargement, I will do a fine needle aspiration."

"Fine," I announced, feeling both relieved that Dr. Loh still felt the lump was fibrocystic and pleased that he was being very thorough by doing an aspiration biopsy.

Then Dr. Loh approached me with a small needle and syringe. He swabbed the lump at the seven o'clock position, inserted the needle, and pulled back the syringe to obtain his specimen. When he was through, I tried to see the syringe contents, but the specimen was away and out of my sight.

Therefore, I blurted to Dr. Loh, "Did the specimen look fine? Is everything all right?"

Dr. Loh nodded his head in assurance and stated, "This continues to be fibrocystic breast condition, and I do not see anything suspicious or problematic."

"I'm glad to hear that, but are you absolutely, 100 percent, sure that everything is fine?" I asked with concern since my breast lump was so large.

Then Dr. Loh smiled, as if embarrassed by my question, and announced very quickly, "Well, if you want a second opinion, I recommend the Lauren Breast Clinic. However, this is benign fibrocystic breast condition."

Immediately, I felt relieved that Dr. Loh held firmly to the benign fibrocystic diagnosis, despite my questioning him. Therefore, I blurted, "I'm so glad you think the lump is fine."

"Yes, well I'd like to see you in three months for a follow-up appointment to see how things are going."

"Fine, Dr. Loh. Thank you for your help."

As I left the office, I was so relieved and happy with the benign diagnosis that I rushed home to phone Isaac with the news. Of course, when I spoke to Isaac he was very pleased with the continued benign diagnosis and told me that is what he suspected.

Then I phoned my mother and my dear friends who had been praying for me. When I told them of my fibrocystic diagnosis, I was both happy and felt a tiny bit foolish for having been so upset over something that was repeatedly benign. Of course, everyone was glad about my good news, and we all thanked God for protecting me.

Following my phone calls, I was exhausted from prior worry over my breast lump. Therefore, I rested a long time on our sofa, while Jay watched television beside me. A few hours later, when Isaac came home from work, I still felt worn-out, so I went straight to bed and slept many long hard hours that night and for the following few nights, making up for lost sleep.

About three days later, after my body and mind finally felt fully rested, I realized that I had never thanked my pastor and his wife for their prayers for my appointment. As I began to dial their number in the mid-afternoon, I suddenly remembered that I did not yet have my fine needle aspiration result. Therefore, I quickly hung up the phone.

The next thing I knew I was dialing Dr. Loh's for the fine needle aspiration report. Naturally, with Dr. Loh's latest diagnosis, I thought that I would only be confirming that my breast lump was benign. After the phone rang for a while, a voice finally answered it and stated, "Hello, this is Dr. Loh's office."

"Hi, this is Robin Gray. I'm calling to get the result of my breast fine needle aspiration from Monday."

"Wait a minute, Robin, and I'll look for the result."

After a few minutes of waiting, I thought the office staff was not very organized. Then as a more minutes passed, during this seemingly eternal wait, my stomach cramped in spasms, wondering if the secretary was actually trying to locate Dr. Loh to give me some kind of bad news.

Finally, the office secretary returned to the phone stating, out of breath, "Hi, Robin, we looked and looked but couldn't find the result. It's not completed yet, but it should be back by tomorrow. We'll give you a call then."

"Oh, okay. Well, thanks. I'll talk to you tomorrow."

A few hours later, at about 3:50 p.m., I was watching a bit of my favorite show, Oprah, when I heard the garage door open. I was somewhat startled, but I figured it was Isaac, home unusually early from work. As I turned off the television to see what was going on, Isaac grimly entered the living room with a sad, solemn look written on his face. Dumb, I did not catch on that he was going to be the bearer of bad news, as I wondered what was going on.

Then he announced in a serious voice, "Robin, look, I got a phone call late this afternoon from Dr. Loh. He said that atypical cells were found on your fine needle aspiration today, and you'll need a lumpectomy, which has been scheduled for one week from now."

"What? I asked wryly. "Are you sure there isn't some kind of mistake? I just spoke with Dr. Loh's office today, and they didn't even have my report. Anyway, how can it be? Dr. Loh has been telling me all along that this is fibrocystic breast condition."

With a dead serious face and sad controlled tone, Isaac slowly announced, "There is no mistake. I just spoke to Dr. Loh about an hour ago. When you called him, he didn't want to give you the bad pathology on the phone, so he called me. He told me the fine needle aspiration was atypical or not normal, and the lump needs to come out."

"Oh my God!" I gasped, throwing my hands over my mouth. In total despair, I dropped into the sofa with suffocating fright.

Then Isaac assured, "You'll be okay. Dr. Loh said that atypical breast cells are not necessarily cancerous. However, the only way to be sure is to get the entire lump out for pathology analysis. I'm so sorry," Isaac conciliatorily muttered.

Once I heard the word "sorry", I fell apart, crying hysterically with my whole body shaking over the harsh blow of bad news. Gradually my loud crying turned into quiet weeping, as I sat on our sofa in a despondent daze for hours. Totally out of my normal composure, Isaac carried out my motherly chores for me. He feed our children supper, cleaned them up, and put them into bed for the night.

The next few days, I was far from my usual self. I could hardly eat due to my nervous stomach and shaky hands. Additionally, I felt physically drained, spacey with fear, and had a hard time focusing on things. Somehow, like a robot, I carried out my necessary household chores and child rearing duties but with a detached heavy-laden mind.

In order to try to cope with my burdens, I read my Bible and fervently prayed to God to protect me and give me peace. I also contacted some dear family members and asked them to pray for me. However, I was still overwhelmed.

Finally, when the weekend arrived, I started to calm down. By then, not only was I adjusting to the idea of surgery, but also my husband was home and encouraging me that a benign diagnosis was still possible. Therefore, I began to feel more hopeful.

Of course, once the weekend was over and my pre-operative appointment arrived on Monday, I was worried again. At least, Isaac's parents came that day to my home to watch Jay, so I could go to Dr. Loh's pre-operative appointment without distraction.

When I finally arrived at Dr. Loh's office, Molly, the usual friendly nurse, led me to the exam room. Unfortunately, the warm air turned coldly sterile when the nurse practitioner entered the exam room, blurting in a shrill voice, "I'm Mrs. Shock, and Dr. Loh has asked me to do a physical on you for surgery. What is your health history?"

"Hi, I'm Robin," I stated, wondering where the kind hellos from Mrs. Shock were. Then I announced, "Back in 1976 I had a rhinoplasty, in 1981 I had kidney stones, and I had three healthy pregnancies with one miscarriage. I don't have any allergies, and I'm not on any medications.

"Okay. What's your extended family's health history?" asked Mrs. Shock.

"Well, I don't know of any current health problems with my siblings or parents. My mom is a retired fitness teacher, and I think she's in good health. My dad still works and seems to be doing well. But both of my grandmothers died of breast cancer."

"What? There is nothing wrong with your parents?"

"Uh, not that I know of."

"What's wrong with you? Are you an orphan or something, not knowing your parents' health history?"

"No, I'm not an orphan. I'm doing the best I can here with the questions. My parents really don't have any major health conditions, at least that I'm aware of," I replied nicely.

"Well, I'm ordering you blood work and a mammogram before the lumpectomy," Mrs. Shock demanded in a drill-sergeant voice.

"A mammogram is going to hurt too much with a lump this size, so do I really need it since the lump is coming out anyway?"

"The mammogram is just routine procedure so the doctor knows what he's dealing with prior to surgery. You do want the surgery?"

"Yes, of course, but I'm afraid this huge lump will hurt when my right breast is compressed during the mammogram," I complained nervously.

"Well, I'll write a prescription for an analgesic; therefore, you can take some pain medication before the mammogram," replied Mrs. Shock.

"Thanks."

"I'd like to assess your breast lump now," announced Mrs. Shock.

I apprehensively reclined back on the exam table and opened my little patient gown to expose my right breast, which contained the lump. Mrs. Shock palpated the lump, as her eyes got large and her face wrinkled up in a frustrated frown. Then she shouted, "That's a huge lump. Why did you let it get so big?"

I was flabbergasted that Mrs. Shock was accusing me of keeping the lump. After all, her boss, Dr. Loh, told me that my breast lump was benign and required no treatment. In fact, I was so appalled that my mouth hung open, and I was speechless.

Then Mrs. Shock continued on scolding, "Now, that's going have to come out, and it is going to leave a huge hole."

"Oh my God!" I muttered in fright as my heart began racing because I could not bear to imagine having a large hole in my chest.

"Yep, this will leave a hole alright with the small breast you have. Anyway, what's wrong--is everybody in your family small-breasted?" asked Mrs. Shock with a snicker.

I was so stunned that Mrs. Shock was in-appropriately interrogating me about the small size of my breasts and about how the surgery would leave me with a huge hole that I wanted to cry. However, I held the tears back, as I knew this insensitive woman would have more ammunition for ridicule.

When the tall probing Mrs. Shock was finally done with her assessment, I raced out of the exam room, right into the reception room, and burst into tears. Molly, the friendly office nurse, rushed up to me, trying to calm me down. I cried to her that the lumpectomy would leave a huge hole in my breast. Then Molly gently assured me that the hole would fill in with new tissue and would look fine. I half believed her enough to stop crying, and I immediately fled to Isaac's office, utterly shaken.

When I got there, Isaac took me back into a private room, as I cried with despair. "Isaac, I can't have my lump cut out. I'm going to look like a freak with a hole in my breast, and how will you ever love me?" I cried.

"Look, Robin, you've got to have the lump out, and we'll fix your breast from there with plastic surgery. I'll take you anywhere in the world you want to have cosmetic surgery. I don't care how much it costs, but you've got to have this lump out."

"I know you're right, Isaac, but it's just so hard to except all this bad news."

"Well, we'll take it one step at a time," encouraged Isaac.

When I got home, I really felt down and worried, thinking I would loose half of my breast. I wondered if Isaac would still really love me the same now that I was going to lose part of my feminine figure. However, when I spoke to Isaac about this, later in the evening, he assured me that he would love me the same and stated that he was never was a boob man anyway. Therefore, I felt better with my sad state of affairs and more prepared to face my surgery.

In fact, the following day, I went to my pre-operative mammogram full of assurance and optimism. However, once the radiologist told me that I had an abnormal mammogram with a suspicious calcification of unknown origin, I got very worried again.

Then, as soon as the appointment was over, I fearfully ran up to Isaac's office, two floors above me in the same building. Of course, Isaac was busy seeing patients, but he stepped out an exam room to speak with me because he could see that I was upset. Then I told him about the mammogram, but he seemed strong and reassured, telling me that everything was going to be okay and that a calcification did not necessarily indicate that my breast lump was cancerous. I was not aware that not all calcifications were harmful, so I calmed down a bit, thinking I still had a chance for a benign lumpectomy.

When I got home, I probably would have been a non-functional mess except I had to hold myself together for my out-of-town houseguests, my parents, who were going to watch my kids while I had surgery. I cleaned the house vigorously, making sure that everything was immaculate, trying to assure everybody and myself that I was holding it together.

Once they arrived, things moved so fast that before I knew it, I was in a hospital room and awaiting surgery. Ironically, my room was on a nursing floor that I had formally worked on when I practiced nursing. In fact, a former co-worker admitted me. At least I felt somewhat familiar with my environment and the people there.

Still, I found it difficult to be a patient that was awaiting surgery and a possible cancer diagnosis. In fact, I was downright scared to death.

Then to make me more nervous, the nurse announced that I would need a breast needle localization procedure in the mammography department prior to surgery. I certainly did not like the idea that my breast was about to be needled prior to surgery.

At least, once I got to mammography, a kind radiologist introduced himself and fully informed me about the localization procedure, which had been unfamiliar to me. He said that he would first place my right breast into the mammogram machine. Next, he instructed that he would insert a sharp narrow wire into my right breast, and anchored it at the calcification shown on the mammogram. Then he assured that the anchored wire would stay put during surgery, enabling the surgeon to locate and remove the suspicious calcified area.

Unfortunately, as the procedure was started, it was every bit as painful as I imagined. First, the machine painfully smashed down my breast and sensitive breast lump. Then, while I was in the mammogram machine, the radiologist injected my breast with lidocaine for numbing. However, the procedure was still extremely painful as the radiologist pushed a thin wire deeply into my breast until the calcification was finally located. Miraculously, once the procedure was finally over, my pain quickly dissipated, and the nurse wheeled me back to my patient room.

About an hour later, my nurse started an intravenous line and carted me off to the Operating Room Holding Room. My stomach cramped, as I worried about possibly having cancer in my breast. While I was in this panicky state, with Isaac by my side, Dr. Loh entered the holding area and approached us with a half smile while he stated, "Do you folks have any last-minute questions?"

"Well, let's just hope everything goes well today," I nervously stated. Then I asked, "How long will the..."

Before I could finish my question, Dr. Loh interrupted, "We'll know the pathology result in a few days."

Great, I thought, *I was going to ask him how long surgery would be.* It was obvious to me what he was thinking about, the pathology, which concerned me.

Before I could worry more, however, I was in the operating room, getting anesthesia. As my mind went out, I prayed that God would protect me.

Sometime later, I awoke in the day surgery unit with intense searing pain across the right side of my chest. The nurse gave me a pill for the pain, which was strong and put me to sleep.

When I awoke, my pain was gone, and I felt comfortable. Therefore, the nurse discharged me and informed me that Dr. Loh would speak to me the following week at my postoperative follow-up appointment.

As I got dressed to leave the hospital, I curiously opened my chest dressing and found a huge ugly hole that covered the entire lower breast from the nipple down. I did not even cry, as Mrs. Shock had more than well prepared me for it.

When I finally got home, in the mid-afternoon, I slept in exhaustion. Later in the evening, I awoke and felt Isaac by my side. As I looked up to him and into his eyes, I suddenly realized he seemed very solemn, so I wondered what was going on. Therefore, I asked,

"Did Dr. Loh say anything to you today about the surgery and what he saw?"

"Well, right after surgery, Dr. Loh said the lump consisted of hard necrotic nodules that could be malignant. At worse, you may need a little radiation."

"Malignant! For God's sake, why didn't you tell me this in the hospital?"

"Well, I didn't want to upset you. Anyway, Dr. Loh said he was 80 percent sure that your breast lump would be benign, even though he saw these hard nodules."

"Great, a 20 percent chance for cancer really upsets and worries me."

"Look, Robin, nobody will know for sure what it is until the pathology comes back, so let's not jump to conclusions. The pathology report should be done in a few days."

"I guess you're right. I just have to hope for the best, but I'm scarred to death."

"Come on, you'll be fine," assured my husband.

"Well, I'm praying you're right, Isaac."

While I waited for my lab report, during the rest of the week and the long weekend, I was so nervous that I could not eat or sleep well. In order to try to calm myself, I prayed frequently, but I was still very anxious.

Finally, when following Monday morning arrived, I was even more nervous, as I expected my test result back that day. Therefore, I kept busy with morning chores to decrease my tension. Suddenly, while I was making the bed in the master bedroom, the phone beside me rang. In a flash, I grabbed it, finding Isaac on the line.

"Hi Robin, I just was in the lab and got your pathology results. I have good and bad news. The bad news is that the lump was cancerous, but the good news is that it's only precancerous and called ductal carcinoma in situ, or DCIS," assured Isaac.

"Oh my God, Isaac!"

"Now don't worry, Robin. I just spoke to Dr. Taylor, who is a fantastic oncologist. He assured me that you have an excellent prognosis with 100 percent cure after treatment. You're lucky it wasn't an invasive cancer, or you'd be getting chemotherapy instead of perhaps just a bit of radiation."

"Radiation?" I muttered nervously.

"Radiation is no big deal," assured Isaac. "Anyway, you may not even need it with a precancerous mass."

"Well, I hope I don't need it," I stated frightfully.

"Robin, you'll need to see and speak to a radiation oncologist. When you call for an appointment, try to get it set up for tomorrow afternoon when I have off from work. I want to be there with you."

"Okay, Isaac. Thanks, I want you to be there too. This is all so scary."

"I know it is, but you'll be fine. I'm sorry to have to tell you all this on the phone, but I didn't want to keep you waiting a minute longer with the pathology result. However, I'm coming home early to be with you…"

When I got off the phone, I cried hysterically for some time. However, I eventually caught on to the idea of the so-called precancerous mass, which did not require chemotherapy and had 100 percent cure rate. I held tightly on to the best part of the diagnosis almost instinctively so I could concentrate on the steep mountain climb ahead of me, and I thanked God for not allowing anything worse.

Later that day, when I was a bit calmer, I called my mother to update her on my pathology result. I gave her the news delicately, and I emphasized the fact that I had a precancerous mass and not an invasive cancer, so she could easily digest it. However, she was immediately angry and yelling, "How could God allow this to happen to my daughter, who has always been such a good Christian girl? You never ran around with guys, smoked, drank, did drugs, or did anything wrong. It's not fair!" Of course, I was surprised that my mom was so angry. I immediately tried to calm her down by telling her that I was going to be fine and lucky to have only a precancerous lump. Thankfully, my assurances finally seemed to settle her.

After that difficult phone call, I managed to phone my sister and a few close friends who had been praying for me. I gave them the news also in the most positive way to ease their acceptance. Funny, I was so busy convincing everybody that I would be okay that I made myself feel a little better about the diagnosis.

When I was finally done with the calls, I took a seat on our sofa and thought about everything. I wondered how breast cancer had formed when Dr. Loh had said the lump was benign for so long.

Bewildered, I assumed he would have a logical explanation at the next visit.

While I was thinking of everything, Dr. Loh's nurse telephoned me, informing me that I needed an appointment with the radiation oncologist. Therefore, I set an appointment up with Dr. Powers, a local radiologist, for the following day, after my appointment with Dr. Loh.

The next day, I arrived at Dr. Loh's office feeling somewhat foggy and lost with my new precancerous diagnosis. At least, the nurse immediately took Jay and I back to the exam room and kindly assured me that things were going to be fine.

Then a moment later, Dr. Loh oddly darted into the exam room, before I had even changed into my patient gown. Therefore, I announced, "Hi, Dr. Loh, I need a minute to get changed into the patient gown that the nurse gave me, so you can check how my incision is healing."

"Okay, I'll be back," he awkwardly replied.

A few minutes later, Dr. Loh nervously walked into the exam room and sheepishly said hello to Jay and I. Then with tired bug-eyes, he quickly and ungracefully muttered, "Nothing is a 100 percent, you know."

Immediately, I thought Dr. Loh was horrible at giving me my precancerous diagnosis. No regrets or an apology was mentioned.

Then he continued rambling on with a fishy look, unable to look me straight in the eye, "You have ductal carcinoma in situ, a precancerous lesion."

"Yes, I know Dr. Loh. Isaac already told me, and he said I was pretty lucky that it was precancerous and not a real invasive cancer."

"Uh-huh. Well, it was a precancerous lesion and uh –big around five centimeters," the old devil said in a soft sheepish voice with his chagrined eyes hanging low.

"Oh?" I muttered in a confused voice, surprised with the huge size of the precancerous mass.

Then Dr. Loh rambled on like a racing train, "You'll need a radiation consultation, which I understand has already been set up. You may choose radiation alone as an option for further treatment, or you may think about having a mastectomy to further decrease cancer recurrence. Furthermore, you may want to consider plastic surgery."

"Plastic surgery—and a mastectomy?" I asked in a stunned voice."

"Yes, these options are possible," replied Dr. Loh.

"Wow, this is overwhelming, but I'll do whatever it takes to get rid of this cancer-- even if that calls for a mastectomy and plastic surgery. Who would do the surgeries?" I asked nervously.

"I can do the mastectomy. The plastic surgery group in town is very good at doing reconstruction of the breasts. However, there is no one-treatment option but various ones. These are all things you'll need to decide personally. You may want just radiation with no further surgery. I suggest that you explore the Internet for various treatment options. Then make your decision. You know there is no rush in your actions with all this. A few weeks delay will not make a difference at this point. You may consider Memorial Sloan-Kettering for care."

"Memorial Sloan-Kettering?" I asked in ignorance.

"It's a world recognized cancer center in New York City," replied Dr. Loh.

"Oh," I stated, still in dazed shock with all of the recommendations and suggestions.

While my mind was spinning, Dr. Loh said, "Let's look at the incision site." He peered at the horizontal five-inch long incision across my chest and announced, "Oh, it looks good. I'd like to see you for another follow-up in two weeks."

"Okay," I replied nervously, still overwhelmed with the various treatment options, and Dr Loh waved good-bye and exited.

Then I dressed in a flash and anxiously darted off in my van to pick up Jay's babysitter, so I could be at my next appointment without a distracting toddler. By the time I finally got the sitter back to my home, Isaac was already home, and my next appointment with the radiation oncologist, Dr. Powers, was approaching quickly.

Therefore, we gave the sitter a few quick instructions. Then we very nervously buzzed off in our van for my oncology appointment. During the drive, I told Isaac I was upset with all of the treatments that Dr. Loh had mentioned at my appointment. Of course, Isaac assured me that I would be okay, but I could tell he was nervous by his fast-paced speech.

When we finally got to the radiation oncology center, we waited quite a long time until the nurse finally took us to an exam room. Then at last, Dr. Powers entered my exam room with a friendly smile and stated, "Hello, Dr. Gray, it's nice to see you here with your wife. Not all spouses are supportive. Robin, I am Dr. Powers and it's nice to meet you. I understand your breast cancer was quite large."

"Hi, Dr. Powers. I can thank Dr. Loh for the huge lump. He informed me several times, over the course of seventeen months, that it was only fibrocystic and could enlarge harmlessly. Now look how I ended up. I just don't understand it. What do you think of him?"

"He's a very good doctor, and I have trusted him to do surgery on my own mother. However, I'm surprised that nothing was done about the enlarging mass. Let's see, according to your initial mammogram, there was no cancer. Now over a year later, you have a calcification. I wish we had a 'Star Track' scanning device that could detect breast cancer earlier.

As I look at your lumpectomy pathology report, five centimeters of your seven-centimeter breast mass was ductal carcinoma in situ. Nothing was cystic in your breast mass. You still have a few unclean margins where cancer still exists. Unclean, cancerous margins are not good because such margins increase the risk of cancer relapse. Normally surgeons like to obtain a clean one-centimeter margin of normal tissue, surrounding the area where the cancer was removed. The goal is to have clean margins to help assure that the cancer has been eradicated and will not reoccur."

"My God, I still have more cancer?" I asked fearfully.

"Yes, but we can treat positive margins with more surgery and/or radiation which removes the cancer and lowers your rate of local or distant cancer recurrence," assured Dr. Powers.

"Oh, I see," I stated.

"Well, Robin, I need to do a physical breast exam now." Then as the doctor palpated my breast, she announced, "Oh, you have quite a bit of disfigurement there. You also have small breasts, which will make more surgery and radiation difficult. Therefore, I suggest that you have a mastectomy, and I recommend you see an oncologist."

"You mean I've got to loose my entire breast?" I gasped.

Isaac hung his mouth open for a moment. Then he began to weep and asked, "Are—are you sure?"

"Yes, I'm sorry, but this is Robin's best option. With a mastectomy, she will obtain an excellent prognosis of nearly 100 percent, and she will not require radiation."

"Oncologist? Mastectomy?" I cried as a tidal wave of tears rolled down my face. The loss of my breast, loss of my health, loss of an early prompt diagnosis, and loss of faith in Dr. Loh finally hit me all at once. Finally, I could see past the thick clouds of deception, revealing the huge mountain of cancerous trouble before me.

As I cried and mourned, Dr. Powers announced, "I'm sorry. I'm done here, but you two can stay as long as you need in this exam room to calm down."

"Thanks," replied Isaac, as I continued to weep bitterly. About ten minutes into our grief, Isaac and I finally calmed down and mustered up the strength to move on.

When we finally got home, I grew very angry with Dr. Loh. Then I said to Isaac, "The seventeen-month fibrocystic diagnosis was a sham, and nothing in the lumpectomy pathology was cystic. Yet, Dr. Loh repeatedly assured me that my breast lump was cystic. I doubt if Dr.

Loh even inserted the needle from my first fine needle aspiration in the correct location. If he did, why wasn't cancer found?"

"I agree that he must have done the fine needle aspiration wrong, if we're now finding out that the same lump in question is cancerous."

"Well, he certainly set me up for the big fall, and he is going to have to answer to me. But, I'm in the battle for my life, at the moment. I'll deal with him later."

The following day, Isaac and I met with my new medical oncologist, Dr. Tayone. He was a very friendly, upbeat oncologist who also happened to be my husband's partner and a family friend for many years. Even so, my husband and I were nervous meeting with him. However, he immediately put us at ease, informing us that I was lucky only to have a precancerous lump. Then he assured us, in a long lengthy conversation, that a mastectomy was my best option for eradicating the unclean margins. He also told me that such surgery would leave me cancer free and without the necessity of chemotherapy. Of course, I was relieved to hear such news.

At the same time, the idea of loosing my breast due to Dr. Loh's late surgical interventions brewed in my head. Instead of a simple lumpectomy with early diagnosis, now I faced a mastectomy. Therefore, I, "Dr. Tayone, what do you think about Dr. Loh's seventeen-month delayed cancer diagnosis?"

"Well, I think it would be hard to prove that Dr. Loh was negligent. We don't even know that the lump was cancerous when you first saw Dr. Loh. Even if it was, how can you prove that, Robin?"

Disappointingly, I replied, "It may be hard to prove, but I know he was negligent. I will never trust him again, and I certainly will be getting out of town for the mastectomy surgery. I'm going to a larger cancer center where there will be outstanding physicians that I can trust."

Chapter Learning Tips

After your diagnostic tests to rule out cancer are done and should you find out that your breast lump is malignant, please be reassured that you have found your cancer as early as possible and have the best chance for an excellent prognosis. The following are a few tips for those who have been diagnosed with breast cancer.

1. Remember the diagnosis of your cancer subtype will determine your treatment. Therefore getting a second pathology opinion on your fine needle aspiration or breast biopsy slides from a breast pathologist will help to make sure that it has been diagnosed correctly and will be treated correctly.

2. Consider larger cancer centers for treatment recommendations and cancer surgeries since larger cancer centers have some of the best and most experienced cancer doctors. The Internet may help you find outstanding cancer centers.

3. Forward your medical records and lab reports to the cancer center where you will be treated.

4. Check with your insurance company to see if they will pay for your treatments.

5. Consider any anti-anxiety medications to help you get through this difficult time.

6. Consider accepting outside assistance with cooking, cleaning, child rearing responsibilities, and so on.

Chapter 4

Treatments and Battle Wounds

To date, there is no perfect cure for cancer. Until there is, treating physicians must continue to seek to diagnose breast cancer as early as possible and treat it immediately and aggressively.

_Breast Cancer a Practical Guide 3rd ed., 2005

My favorite time of year was blossoming on the mountain at my home in 2002, but I hardly knew it. My eyes were buried in preparing for the biggest trip, the journey to save my life. Day and night, I obsessively read multiple breast cancer Internet websites and breast cancer books, determined not to be mislead by physicians again and to beat cancer.

I was so focused on learning how to survive and arranging treatments that I had little time for little Jay. Unfortunately, Jay did not take to my stress well. He regressed in his toilet training, and he started to stutter. I felt terrible that he was burdened by my medical nightmare. In order to reduce his stress and be more available to him during the day, I began doing most of my research after he went to bed. I felt drained, being the midnight owl, but at least Jay's behavior slowly improved.

Through my midnight madness of surfing the net, I learned that the Johns Hopkins Hospital in Baltimore, MD and Memorial Sloan-Kettering Cancer Center in Manhattan, New York, both had outstanding breast cancer treatment programs and were only four hours from my home. At first, I favored the Johns Hopkins Hospital for care since I had worked there years earlier as an intensive care nurse and knew the hospital and area. However, I eventually spoke with an acquaintance of mine who had gone to Memorial Sloan-Kettering Cancer Center in Manhattan, New York, for a mastectomy and she had excellent results there with her breast surgeon, Dr. Jeanne Petrek. Naturally, I could not resist a personal recommendation, so I arranged doctor appointments at the distant cancer center with Dr. Petrek. At the same time, Isaac arranged for his parents to watch our kids while we were out of town in Manhattan.

When the day of the consults finally arrived in Manhattan, Isaac and I nervously found ourselves an hour early at Dr. Petrek's office. Immediately, I noticed a large waiting room that was full of women at least ten to twenty years older than I was. Therefore, I felt somewhat angry, being younger with breast cancer, and I wondered what I had done to deserve it. Upset, I ran in the bathroom and freshened up my lipstick to make myself feel better.

When I got back to the waiting area, Isaac told me an older woman in the waiting room had came up to him and told him that his wife would be okay. Consequently, I felt calmer, knowing that an encouraging angel was among us.

Then in a slightly rattled state, I completed a ton of medical history forms, asking me about such things as breastfeeding history and birth control use. As I completed them, I found my mind drifting into the past...

I remembered when I first became scared of breast cancer, at eight years old, when my paternal grandmother flashed her chest to me, revealing her ugly mastectomy scar.

I remembered that every time I bathed from then on, I frightfully felt for breast lumps.

I remembered finding a lump in my right breast when I was about ten years old and showing it to my parents, but they only said it was a developing breast bud.

I remembered, soon after that, having a crazy fifth-grade boy classmate grabbing my unprotected developing right breast with pliers while I was innocently standing outside at the playground.

I remembered that my right breast never grew much more after that and my left breast was always a little bigger, but I never thought it would harm me, though I did feel awkward.

I remembered, in early marriage, I was fearful that birth control pills could cause breast cancer; however, my gynecologist said that the pills were harmless. Therefore, I took them for several months until we decided to start a family.

I remembered, once my kids were born, that I happily breastfed, believing, as the medical community preached, that it may help to prevent breast cancer.

I remembered how often I thought of and feared breast cancer throughout my life, more than any other woman that I knew.

Now I had breast cancer. How ironic that no amount of worrying had prevented my breast cancer diagnosis. Just like my grandmother, I had to face an ugly mastectomy. I hated the idea, but I was beginning to accept it, in hopes that it would save my life.

As I waited to see Dr. Petrek, I opened a cancer treatment booklet that I had brought with me and began to read full force with a mindset to win the long battle ahead. Three long hours into my laborious readings, Dr. Petrek's nurse finally shouted out my name to see the doctor next. Excited, Isaac and I darted back to Dr. Petrek's exam room, but there was more endless waiting. Therefore, I began wondering if I had chosen the right cancer center.

Finally, Dr. Petrek's tall, slender middle-aged body busily bustled into the exam room where we waited. She kindly apologized for her delay with a magnetic smile. Then she got down to business and began to examine my breasts. As she carefully palpated them, she complimentarily stated, "You're thin like a Fifth-Avenue model. You certainly don't have enough fat for the autologous fat breast implant breast reconstruction."

I laughed shyly at the doctor's kind comments.

Then she continued on stating, "The saline breast implant type of reconstruction is what you need. You'll look great with the implants after your mastectomy."

"Do you definitely feel the mastectomy is required, Dr. Petrek?" I asked inquisitively.

"Oh yes, your pre-cancer was too large and hasn't left you with enough breast tissue for any other surgical choice. Furthermore, due to the large size of your DCIS, a higher risk for lymph node invasion exists. So you'll also need a sentinel lymph node dissection as well."

"What, a sentinel node dissection?" I asked puzzled.

"Yes, a sentinel node surgery will help to see if your cancer has spread."

"Cancer spread?" I nervously asked.

"Well, the odds are very much in your favor that there has been no cancer spread into your lymph nodes," assured Dr. Petrek.

Then I asked, "Would any risk of cancer in my lymph nodes have existed if I hadn't suffered a seventeen-month delayed cancer diagnosis?"

Suddenly Dr. Petrek grew silent, suggesting her reluctance to comment. Then she finally confessed, "It's rare to see a cancer this large in a young woman. I am very concerned over the large size of your cancer and the aggressive cytology of comedo necrosis."

"Well, my breast lump was very small when I first saw my local surgeon. He repeatedly told me that the lump was only fibrocystic, even as it enlarged over the seventeen-month period when I saw him. He also told me that the brown nipple secretions from my right breast were normal to have in fibrocystic breast condition. Now I bet that nipple drainage was an ominous sign. I'm in this predicament due to his misdiagnosis," I announced defiantly.

Dr. Petrek reservedly nodded. Then she continued to look at the 2002 lumpectomy pathology report and shook her head in negation, stating, "I'm concerned about the language in this pathology report from a legal standpoint. It says that 'frankly invasive disease' was not present. I think we better check this out just to be sure you only have pure DCIS."

"Well, I brought my pathology slides today for a second opinion."

"Great, I'll have the New York City Pathology Group look at these for a second pathology opinion. I'll let you know the results. Let's also set a surgical date now. My schedule is busy. I am going on vacation, and the soonest I have is the beginning of June."

Then Isaac said, "How about June fifth? That's a perfect date for me. I happen to have vacation during that time."

"But is it okay to wait three more weeks to clear positive margins, Dr. Petrek?" I asked nervously.

"Yes, it should be fine and not harm you.

"In that case, I guess I will see you in a few more weeks for surgery." I replied.

Then Dr. Petrek stated, "I would like you to schedule an ultrasound and mammogram appointment here in Manhattan with Dr. Kolb or Dr. Lichy before your surgery."

"Oh, do I need both those tests again since I just had them?"

"Yes, these tests will help me in surgery. Here's an article by Dr. Lichy and Dr. Kolb. It explains the importance of ultrasound in finding breast cancer in young women. Mammography is only 70 percent accurate in young pre-menopausal women in their thirties because their female hormones often clouds the mammogram film and can obscure cancer."

"Good grief, my initial radiologist, Dr. Covington, never told me that mammography wasn't accurate in young women. Maybe that's why I had a negative mammogram when I really had a cancerous lump. At least I did have the ultrasound, but that didn't find my cancer either. I wonder why not?"

Dr. Petrek shrugged her shoulders and got quiet quickly, as if she did not want to talk about my misdiagnosis. Therefore, I did not press the issue.

Then Dr. Petrek said, "You'll need to arrive a few days before surgery for general preoperative testing and for the pre-operative sentinel lymph node blue dye injection. That dye procedure will help map out your lymph nodes and allow me to find them during your surgery. You can arrange all these tests with my secretary."

After Dr. Petrek had exited the exam room, Isaac announced, "She was impressive. I'm very pleased she's going to treat you aggressively with the mastectomy and sentinel node dissection."

"Yep Isaac, I am too. She offered me a lot more than Dr. Loh ever did. It looks like our long wait for the good Dr. Petrek was worthwhile."

The next day, we met Dr. Cordeiro, the plastic surgeon, at his midtown Manhattan office. Without wait, the nurse took us to the exam room where Dr. Cordeiro, a small built man, introduced himself. He spoke rapidly, like a car salesperson, about the various options for breast reconstruction. When his speech was over, it was apparent that the best method of reconstruction for me was bilateral saline breast implants, which would offer me some overall bust enlargement and breast symmetry. Of course, I liked the idea that I would be getting an increase in breast size. I was excited for something uplifting at last. Furthermore, the saline implants seemed very safe. Therefore, I immediately signed the consent form for the surgery, which was scheduled with my mastectomy.

When we were finally done with the appointments, we went back to our fancy Marriott Hotel and relaxed on the beds. Then I teased Isaac that he might like my new breast enhancing implants because I may look sexier than ever. Then Isaac assured me that he liked my body the way it was, as he kissed me like a wild man in love.

About three days after we returned from New York City, I received a phone call from Dr. Petrek. She informed us that the pathologist had contacted her and reported no invasive breast cancer in my breast lumpectomy slides. However, Dr. Petrek informed me that I still had a 2 percent risk of invasion in the axillary lymph nodes, which was possible due to the large size of the DCIS.

Of course, even a small risk of cancer invasion outside of the breast to regional lymph nodes worried me. I was nervous and extremely frustrated at Dr. Loh for allowing my precancerous breast lump to enlarge. Isaac was upset too. He wondered why Dr. Loh had misdiagnosed me and why he had not apologized.

About this time, my husband was working at the hospital and he ran into Dr. Loh. Of course, Isaac told the negligent surgeon that I was very angry about the misdiagnosis and that I deserved an apology phone call. To Isaac's surprise, Dr. Loh defended himself, indicating that he had followed a breast assessment algorithm or guide, which verified his actions.

As the days passed, I still did not hear from Dr. Loh for an apology. I suspected that I would never hear from him again. However, a few days before my surgery at the Memorial Sloan-Kettering Cancer Center, I heard the phone ring. I picked it up in a causal calm manner until I heard who was on the receiver...

"Hello, Robin, this is Dr. Loh. I'm just calling to wish you luck with your mastectomy at Memorial Sloan-Kettering."

"What? Good luck? Well, I appreciate that, but I'm not just having a mastectomy but also a sentinel lymph node dissection," I stated with frustration.

"I don't see the need for that, in a case like yours, with just DCIS (ductal carcinoma in situ)," Dr. Loh defended.

"Well, my breast surgeon from the Memorial Sloan-Kettering said I needed the sentinel node dissection surgery because my DCIS was so large that a risk for invasion into my lymph node and elsewhere was very possible." I snapped with frustration.

"That's very aggressive treatment," Dr. Loh stated.

"It's about time someone treated me aggressively. Why did you always falsely assure me that my breast lump was fibrocystic breast condition? My lump was cancerous and required immediate removal. Why did you give me such cavalier care?"

"Oh no, I didn't give you cavalier treatment, not at all. I did the same for you that I do for all of my patients," Dr. Loh defended.

"Really, then what went wrong? After my recent research, I find you should have immediately done a biopsy on my breast lump early on, but you waited until four months to do a fine needle aspiration biopsy. Not only did you delay my fine needle aspiration, but you never told me that it was subject to a high rate of error and that the core or excisional biopsies are more accurate than the fine needle aspiration for detecting cancer."

"Well, I did the best I could to help you."

"Really? Well, I told you that the lump was enlarging at the six-month follow-up. You assured it was only benign fibrocystic condition, using an office ultrasound and breast exam. Now I learn that those tests can't definitely rule out cancer. Why didn't you know that?"

"I did everything I could to properly diagnose you. I don't know what went wrong here," whispered Dr. Loh sheepishly. "This kind of thing has never happened to me before."

"Well, I just hope you don't misdiagnose other women with breast lumps."

"Yes, oh yes, I'll be more careful," Dr. Loh assured brightly.

When I hung up the phone, my hands shook, as the phone conversation was upsetting. However, I let my emotions drop quickly in order to organize for the out-of-town surgeries.

As I planned everything, I was stressfully overwhelmed with a billion things to do all at once. I was busy making childcare arrangements, hotel reservations, educating myself on breast cancer treatments, and taking care of my three young children.

To add to my burdens, my health insurer informed me that my plan would only cover 20 percent of eighty thousand dollars worth of surgical bills at the Memorial Sloan-Kettering Cancer Center. I tried desperately to change the plan prior to surgery. However, I was not allowed to change on such short notice. At least Isaac and I were able to obtain a huge second mortgage to cover my medical expenses.

As my surgery date approached, my parents arrived from Baltimore, Maryland, to my home in upstate New York like winged angels. They brought me gifts, food, and hands ready to help with household chores and childcare. Thankfully, my kids loved the attention from their grandparents, and were peaceful as Isaac and I left for my surgery in Manhattan, New York.

Once we finally got down to the big city, we checked into an economy hotel, and I began my many preoperative hospital tests over the course of the next two days. This included routine blood work, chest X-ray, EKG, the sentinel node mapping with blue dye injection into my breast, and a preoperative breast ultrasound.

Interestingly during my breast ultrasound, Dr. Lichy, a world-renowned radiologist in breast imaging, commented on my delayed cancer diagnosis. He informed me that Dr. Loh should have done the more reliable core biopsy for an enlarging lump, not a fine needle aspiration. Of course, this only made me more frustrated with Dr. Loh.

When we got back to our Manhattan hotel, I cried to Isaac that the cancer had better not be in my lymph nodes, or I would have to sue Dr. Loh. Isaac scolded me for bringing up such matters, as if it would curse my outcome. I figured he was right, so I pleaded with God for no cancer spread. Desperate, I even told God that I would forgive Dr. Loh if my lymph nodes were free of cancer.

The following morning I felt overwhelmed with the thought of losing my breast while I awaited surgery in the operating room waiting suite. I prayed repeatedly for peace, but I felt like a caged little agitated sheep, just before the slaughter.

Finally, after several hours of insufferable waiting for surgery, an anesthesiologist wheeled me into the operating room. Then my breast surgeon, Dr. Petrek, and plastic surgeon, Dr. Cordiero, beautifully wove my mastectomy, my sentinel node dissection, and part of my breast reconstruction for my permanent transformation.

Hours later, I awoke in the recovery room with a nurse shouting that it was 8:30 p.m. and I should be awaking. However, I felt half-dead from anesthesia, nauseated, and was unable respond to her. While I was in this horrible state, Dr. Petrek visited me, ecstatically shouting in my ear that my surgery went well and my lymph nodes were free of cancer. I was happy to hear such news, but lacked the energy to open my eyes and express my gratitude. Then I drifted off into oblivion.

A couple of hours later, I awoke in a drowsy state inside my new patient room with heavy pain across my chest and arm. Thankfully, a kind nurse gave me a patient control assist (PAC) button, explaining that I could push it and receive a controlled dose of morphine into my intravenous line anytime I wanted it. Of course, I hit the button a bunch of times, hoping to rid myself of my explosive arm pain. The morphine drugged my mind and dragged me off to some place where I was too weak to respond to anything.

By the next morning, I awoke fully with crushing arm pain at six a.m. Scared, I kept my arm still as I prayed for relief.

Finally, the plastic surgeon's Nurse Practitioner visited me at morning rounds, and I told her about my arm pain. To my surprise, she informed me that arm movement would actually decrease my arm discomfort. She also taught me a few postoperative arm exercises, explaining to me they should be done frequently throughout the day to promote healing and prevent arm contracture. Reluctantly, I did the exercises, which, to my surprise, actually did reduce my arm pain and stiffness.

A day later, I was getting around better without so much pain. Therefore, Dr. Petrek discharged me from the hospital with antibiotics and analgesics. As we drove out of the city and back to my home, four hours away, I cried because I was so thankful to be alive and to have my surgical ordeal behind me.

During my recuperation back at home, I had plenty of support from my family and friends. My parents were angels and staying with me at my house to look after my three kids. In addition, it seemed like everybody, from town and out-of-town was sending me food to nourish me back to health.

Several days into my recuperation, I noticed that my surgical site was healing well, and my spirits were optimistic for a bright cancer free future. I knew I had been through a lot, and I was ready to enjoy life. Unfortunately, about this time the phone rang with some bad news.

"Hello Robin, this is Dr. Petrek. Your mastectomy only contained DCIS, a precancerous mass, which is good, but you had microscopic cancer cells in your first lymph node."

"Oh no!" I cried. "I thought you told me in the recovery room that my lymph nodes were free of cancer."

"Well, your lymph nodes were free of cancer on frozen section pathology. However, on a more thorough analysis, your first sentinel lymph node was positive for a micro-metastasis by a new monoclonal antibody chemical staining called immunohistochemistry. Now the immunohistochemical test, which is sometimes called the IHC test, is very accurate and sensitive for the smallest amounts of cancer. In your case, it's detecting very scant areas of cancer in your first lymph node. To be precise, the pathologist found exactly thirty-two cancer cells in your node. Consequently, this is a clear indication that cancer has spread beyond your breast. Therefore, you will need chemotherapy. Unfortunately, your survival is probably now decreased about 15 percentage points. However, chemotherapy could improve this decreased survival by 30 percent to leave you with a 10 percent decreased survival instead of 15 percent. I highly suggest chemotherapy which could not only decrease your risk of recurrence but delay a cancer recurrence, if it does occur."

Suddenly, I felt like the wind had just been knocked out of me, and I was suffocating. I gasped for air and heard Isaac, who was listening on another phone next to me, quietly sobbing. Then I somehow managed to nervously ask, "Are you sure there isn't a mistake? Are you sure these are real cancer cells?"

"Oh yes, the IHC test is very accurate and sensitive. You had a very large DCIS. It appears that somewhere-- it did invade."

"Oh no," I cried with horror.

"I'm sorry," consoled Dr. Petrek. However, I do think chemotherapy will help. I suggest you contact the oncology department here as soon as possible for a consult."

"Will I lose my long hair?" I cried, wondering how I could manage to sacrifice another feminine attribute after just losing my breast.

"Robin, there are various chemotherapy regimens, and some less aggressive than others, causing only minimal hair loss. However, I don't know what the oncologist will recommend for you, but wish you the best."

As I hung up the phone, my mind exploded with anger, and I screamed, "Isaac, for God's sake, why did you send me to that idiot, Dr. Loh? He allowed my cancer to spread!"

Immediately, poor Isaac hunched over, crying hysterically and ran to my mother in the basement. At the same time, I ran outside and into our backyard woods like wild fire, intoxicated with miserable grief. I felt cursed, and I knew the old dammed devil had his hand in it. In anger, I ran about in the woods until I was exhausted. Then I wandered back home and apologized to Isaac for the crossfire that should have been aimed at Dr. Loh. Kindly, Isaac forgave me.

Several days later, I still felt horrible, and I had not fully adjusted to the thought of chemotherapy. While I was in this agitated state, the phone rang, and I picked it up.

"Hi, Robin, this is Dr. Petrek. How are you?" she asked like an angel.

"Hi, Dr. Petrek, it's good to hear from you. I am feeling a bit better physically, but emotionally it's hard. I don't like the idea of chemotherapy. You know, I really wonder if chemotherapy is necessary since by traditional pathological staining I would have been node negative and not required chemotherapy. Are you sure the IHC test is accurate and is able to predict a worst cancer prognosis?"

"Robin, there are no prognostic studies done yet to verify the prognostic significance of a micro-metastasis in a lymph node. However, I would predict that your prognosis is not the near 100 percent that is usually seen with DCIS. Now, if your cancer has spread, a cancer recurrence could occur soon or years from now, if it does happen. I know chemotherapy has collateral damage, but I really do think it is your wisest choice. You don't want a relapse."

"Of course, I don't want to have cancer come back. I have kids that I need to be here for. Don't worry. I'll make the oncology consult appointment."

Before I knew it, I was back at the Memorial Sloan-Kettering Cancer Center, in early July, seeing Dr. Fornier, a breast cancer oncologist. She stated that although no one knew the exact prognostic significance of a micro-metastasis, she believed my prognosis was lowered by 12-15 percent and that I required six months of CMF or cyclophosphamide, methotrexate and 5-flurouracil chemotherapy. Immediately, I was upset by her recommendation, and I fell silent. Kindly, she tried to make me feel better by assuring me that my prognosis was good, which made me calm down.

When I got back home, I visited my local oncologist, Dr. Taylor, to see what he thought of the new chemotherapy recommendations from Memorial Sloan-Kettering Cancer Center. He supported some of Dr. Fornier's CMF recommendations, commenting that the other chemotherapy regimen for breast cancer, AC (Adriamycin/Cytoxan), had even worse side effects with a 5 percent chance of causing permanent cardiac damage. Then he stated CMF was much safer with only a 1 percent risk of leukemia and that my cancer recurrence risk far outweighed the 1 percent risk. Of course, the writing was on the wall to do chemotherapy.

Finally, by the end of August, I was starting my first of six intravenous chemotherapy treatments at Isaac's office with Dr. Taylor, a local oncologist. The first treatment was a family affair with my three young sons and husband with me to help me initiate my dreaded journey. As I received my chemotherapy, we prayed for God to protect me.

While I suffered with poisonous treatments, I got mad all over again at Dr. Loh. I knew my struggling was due to his error, so I angrily called a local lawyer to sue my doctor. However, this lawyer revealed that most local lawyers would not be interested in my case against a local physician.

Undiscouraged, I contacted a few other attorneys via the Internet who were in another town. One of those attorneys, Mr. Web, sounded very experienced in breast cancer litigation. We spoke on the phone a few times about my case until he revealed that my lawsuit case would not be settled for five to seven years and that would be preferred, allowing me more time for a recurrence and larger settlement. Of course, I didn't take his pessimistic greediness well, and I immediately dropped him.

Finally, my husband gave me a recommendation for another lawyer, Attorney Torn. When I contacted Mr. Torn, I was impressed by his experience in breast cancer litigation, and he seemed interested in my case. Therefore, I signed a retainer agreement with him. Then, a few weeks later, Attorney Torn sent me a huge packet of my medical records pertaining to my misdiagnosis, including my mammogram report, fine needle aspiration reports, lumpectomy hospitalization, and medical notes from my multiple visits with Dr. Loh.

I immediately read Dr. Loh's records with great interest. When I was done, I was shocked to learn that he never kept a growth record of my breast lump, and he documented that my breast lump was only a thickening of tissue when it was indeed a distinct hard lump. Furthermore, he repeatedly documented a fibrocystic diagnosis. His documentation, at least to me, immediately verified his sloppy medical practices and negligence.

Irritated with Dr. Loh's practices, I phoned my attorney, begging him to sue Dr. Loh as soon as possible. However, my attorney informed me it would take him months to read my entire medical record before he would be able to sue Dr. Loh. Therefore, I went along with the long analysis, thinking there was no great rush to start litigation.

During the next several days, I had the opportunity to review the rest of my multiple medical records related to my misdiagnosis while Isaac was at work, including my initial mammogram report from November 2000. I had never seen the written report, but I figured it would say exactly what I had been told verbally from my radiologist. However, I was shocked when I read that my mammogram report was marked Category IV, Suspicious for Malignancy, based on the radiologist's physical exam. Additionally, the report stated that the lump required a surgical biopsy, if it did not resolve.

Immediately, I was extremely angry that my radiologist, Dr. Covington, failed to tell me of the suspicious report or of the need for a surgical biopsy. He only told me that my mammogram and ultrasound were normal and that I only required long-term follow-up with a surgeon. Furious, I wondered why Dr. Covington did not communicate the bad report to me, especially when I was screaming during the exam with him, "Is my breast lump cancerous?" Furthermore, I wondered why Dr. Covington would not have recommended an immediate biopsy for something that he thought was suspicious for cancer. Surely, an immediate biopsy should have determined that my breast lump was cancerous and required immediate surgical removal.

As I thought about everything, I hoped Isaac would have some answers for me about the bad report, which I never knew about. Later that night, once my husband was home from work, I questioned him.

"Isaac, I just got my initial mammogram report from November 18, 2000 in the mail today from my lawyer, and it says 'Suspicious for Malignancy'. Dr. Covington and Dr. Loh never told me that! In addition, why didn't you tell me about the bad report either? I wanted that mammogram report immediately-- that's why you ordered it as soon as possible. Outrageously, it took me over two years to get the real report! Didn't you have a copy of that report that you could have shown me?"

"Look, I only got your mammogram report after you saw Dr. Loh, You did have a normal mammogram and ultrasound, according to Dr. Covington's verbal and written report. However, based on Dr. Covington's physical exam of your lump, he documented that he felt it was suspicious for cancer. I guess that's why he sent you to the surgeon, who was the ultimate clinical authority on clinical breast exam."

"Well, I wish you had shown me this report. Furthermore, I wish the radiologist had been candid with me when I asked him if the lump was cancerous. Surely, he should have told me that he felt my breast lump was suspicious for cancer based on his clinical breast exam, but he failed to mention this important information. He should be sued," I announced defiantly.

"Yes, Dr. Covington should have told you. However, he still made the appropriate surgical referral. Therefore, nobody will see him as guilty when he did pass the case to the surgeon, Dr. Loh."

"I guess you're right. It may be difficult to convict Dr. Covington legally. However, if I had known that Dr. Covington thought the lump was suspicious for cancer based on his clinical breast exam, then maybe I would have questioned Dr. Loh's benign diagnosis and gotten a second surgical opinion."

"You did ask Dr. Loh about a second opinion, but he told you not to worry about that and assured you that he knew what he was doing and that your breast lump was not suspicious for cancer."

"That's true, Isaac."

"Well, he didn't back down from himself because he was the clinical authority for breast assessment. He should have known more than the radiologist about clinical breast assessment, but he didn't," stated Isaac with disgust.

"Right, he didn't know anything. He told me that my breast lump was benign fibrocystic condition when it was cancerous and when his colleague, the radiologist, clearly reported in his notes that it was suspicious for cancer."

"You're right. Dr. Loh didn't know what he was doing. It just gets me mad that I never saw him make a mistake until my wife needed care. Robin , I am sorry about the whole thing and that my colleagues let us down."

"Yes, they sure did," I agreed in exhaustion, figuring I had better save my energy for healing and chemotherapy treatments.

As days moved forward, I attended my monthly chemotherapy sessions with three-year-old, Jay, by my side. The initial sessions only cramped my stomach.

However, as the sessions progressed into the autumn and the toxicity of chemotherapy accumulated in my body, I had nausea and vomiting for a few days following chemotherapy. Worse than that, my very thick hair began to fall out in clumps all over the place, leaving me with long dry stringy lifeless hair.

By my last chemotherapy session in Dec. 2002, I felt worn out and ripped apart at the seams as if a nuclear explosion had gone off. I was slashed across the chest with a long red scar, was thinner than ever with half my hair gone, and I was starting to suffer from chemotherapy induced menopausal hot flushes. To make matters worse, the cold chill air of winter irritated my surgical arm and breast, giving me stabbing phantom pain. Determined to fight it all, I made the best of things, putting on a bright happy smile for my kids, while I hoped that one day my body would feel normal again.

As the weeks passed, however, my hopes for normalcy were somewhat dampened at my January medical follow-up appointment when I learned from my oncologist that I should consider taking an oral anti-estrogen drug called tamoxifen. The thought of tamoxifen frightened me, as I read it could cause intense hot flashes and rare cases of ovarian cancer. I certainly wasn't happy with the side effects, and I wondered if I really needed the drug.

Therefore, I researched tamoxifen extensively to see what its benefits were. From my research, it appeared that tamoxifen worked by starving estrogen sensitive breast cancer cells to death via blocking the estrogen receptor, thus, decreasing cancer recurrence. At the same time, tamoxifen would be ineffective in invasive breast cancer that would not be sensitive to estrogen.

Oddly, it appeared that tamoxifen was always indicated for ductal carcinoma in situ, DCIS, regardless of estrogen status. However, I had a gut feeling that my DCIS was not estrogen sensitive since I had the rarer type of DCIS, comedo, which I learned was usually hormonal negative and not estrogen sensitive. Therefore, I deducted that an anti-estrogen like tamoxifen would not benefit me.

Naturally, I wanted to be sure of my deductions. Specifically, I wanted to know if my tumor was estrogen/progesterone sensitive. However, my oncologist did not want to do the hormone test on my tumor because he thought that all DCIS should get tamoxifen, regardless of hormonal status.

However, what my oncologist was telling me did not appear logical, and I really wanted to know the estrogen sensitivity of my breast lumpectomy. Therefore, I tenaciously called the Cedar's Hospital pathology department one day and asked to speak to a pathologist about estrogen/progesterone tumor testing. A few minutes later a female voice softly spoke.

"Hi, this is Dr. Lyon."

"Oh hi, Dr. Lyon, this is Robin Gray. I believe we've met before. I'm Dr. Isaac Gray's wife." As I spoke, an image of the model thin Asian woman, Dr. Lyon, formed in my head. I recalled having met her years earlier at, of all places, Dr. Loh's house when he had a mid-winter medical brunch with local doctors and their spouses.

"Oh, Dr. Isaac Gray's wife? Hold on a minute, and let me get your record while I go into my private office." A few moments later, Dr. Lyon announced, "Hi, I'm back."

"Good, I hope I'm not disturbing you, but I did have a few questions for you."

"Oh? How are you? I heard about your breast cancer," Dr. Lyon blurted.

"I'm doing okay. I've just finished chemotherapy, and it's been rough fighting breast cancer with small children. I wouldn't have required chemotherapy if it weren't for the surgeon's seventeen-month delayed diagnosis. Isaac and I are very disappointed with Dr. Loh. I guess we chose the wrong doctor."

"Oh, no, he's a very good doctor," Dr. Lyon persuaded.

"Well, something went wrong in my case. When he did his fine needle aspiration, he missed my cancer. Recently, I read on the Internet that the core biopsy is a safer sampling method with less error than the fine needle aspiration that Dr. Loh performed on me. What do you think?"

"Yes, core biopsies are better, more accurate, and just about all the breast biopsies we get are core," Dr. Lyon assured.

"Well, then why did I get the riskier fine needle aspiration procedure, particularly when most get the core?" I cried.

Then in a whisper Dr. Lyon confided, "You didn't get the core because you're so young."

"Oh, so if I had been older, my breast lump would have been taken more seriously by Dr. Loh? Well, that really makes me angry. Anyway, this isn't your problem. I'm so sorry to be carrying on so. I called to see if a pathologist at your lab could do an estrogen and progesterone study on my breast cancer tissue block from my lumpectomy surgery last spring?"

"Yes, we can get the test done for you via an outside lab," assured Dr. Lyon.

"Good, I believe you have my tissue lumpectomy block. So would you mind sending a sample of my block out for the test?"

"Yes, I can do that."

"Thanks, Dr. Lyon, I appreciate your help, and I hope to hear from you soon."

Sure enough, a few weeks later, I received the estrogen sensitivity test back and learned that my tumor was estrogen negative. Therefore, I figured the anti-estrogen drug, tamoxifen, would not help lower a cancer recurrence. In order to verify my deductions, I forwarded my medical questions and history to Dr. Leroy Parker, a breast oncologist, from the esteemed Dana Farber Cancer Center in Boston, Massachusetts, via of an expensive out-of-pocket Internet e-mail consult.

The doctor immediately responded back with a detailed medical consult e-mail note and phone call, informing me that tamoxifen was not necessary. He cited a very recent study that indicated that tamoxifen would not decrease a cancer relapse from estrogen negative

DCIS. Furthermore, he stated that another new study showed tamoxifen would not prevent a contra-lateral breast cancer since new cancers are usually of the same hormonal status. Assured by the expert, I immediately resigned from taking the dreaded unnecessary medication, tamoxifen.

Finally, I thought things were starting to go my way since I didn't need tamoxifen. I was on cloud nine, figuring nothing could get me down now. However, about that time, the phone rang with some disappointing news...

"Hello, Robin , this is Attorney Torn. I have just finished reading over your medical records. I think the case against Dr. Loh would be challenging to prove since the surgeon did order a fine needle aspiration biopsy that turned out negative."

"What about the six-month follow-up after the fine needle aspiration when I saw Dr. Loh? He did nothing but a lame ultrasound for an enlarging lump! However, recently I learned that he should have done a core or excisional biopsy for a lump that persisted and continued to grow," I cried.

"Well, by the time of your six-month follow-up appointment, the cancer was probably advanced enough not to significantly change the end result of your seventeen-month delayed diagnosis," announced Attorney Torn.

"What?" I cried. "I can't believe what you are telling me. I know Dr. Loh is guilty. I don't think you really understand the medical negligence in this case. I've read recently that the fine needle aspiration he performed was not very reliable because it had a 10% error rate, but he never informed me about that. Furthermore, I believe my pre-cancer would not have invaded and spread to my lymph node if Dr. Loh had diagnosed it sooner."

"I'm sorry, I don't agree with you—Dr. Loh is not guilty. Furthermore, I think that I understand this case well enough, and I don't appreciate your comment that I don't understand the medial aspects of this case. Our personalities DO NOT match, and I suggest you find a new attorney!" scolded Attorney Torn.

"What, are you dumping me?" I cried.

"Well, I may be able to refer you to a colleague of mine who might proceed with this case. However, I must resign from this case since we don't see eye to eye, and I will be mailing you a bill."

"That won't be necessary. I'm capable of finding an attorney supportive of me. Goodbye!" I announced in frustration.

Once I got off the phone, I cried bitterly. Moreover, I felt discouraged at my failing attempts to find a good attorney. I was exhausted, trying to make Dr. Loh accountable for his errors, and I wondered if I should cut my losses.

However, several days later, I somehow got the energy and nerve to contact another attorney experienced in breast cancer litigation that I found on the Internet. He was from Philadelphia and seemed extremely interested in my case, stating that Dr. Loh was negligent. Therefore, I quickly forwarded him my medical records.

Unfortunately, weeks later, he informed he could not take my case either, being so geographically distant from me when the case would not generate enough money for him. Therefore, he forwarded my records to an attorney closer to me.

Within a week, I heard from the new referral attorney. However, he said my case would be hard to prove since it was my fault for getting cancer. I could hardly believe this lawyer's cold accusations, and I immediately dropped the attorney and wondered why I was wasting my time on a lawsuit.

About this time, a friend of mine gave me the phone number of her friend's mother who had recently won a breast cancer lawsuit. I called this woman and got a great referral from her attorney, Mr. Rich, who won her case.

When I called Mr. Rich, he was very nice and thought I had a great case. Therefore, I sent Mr. Rich my medical records, figuring I had nothing to lose. Immediately, the attorney responded back, very optimistically informing me that I had an excellent case. Ecstatic, I agreed to meet him in late March 2003 for a consult.

A few days after I spoke with him, I went to the public library, found some lawsuit books, and began to read a little about medical litigation, thinking it may help me win my medical lawsuit. As I read, I was surprised to learn that a defendant could exonerate himself if another person was not sued but was also guilty in the same malpractice case. I thought this was interesting, but I figured no one but Dr. Loh was at fault in my case.

Then a few weeks later, Isaac brought a very interesting article to my attention from one of his recently published medical journals. It was called, "Causes of Physician Delay in the Diagnosis of Breast

Cancer" by Dr. Goodson and Dr. Moore from the *Archives of Internal Medicine* 2002: pages-1343-1348. It discussed how to avoid a breast misdiagnosis, of all things. Immediately, I wished we had seen the article prior to my own delayed diagnosis, and I paused, wondering if I should torture myself by reading the article. All too curious, I read it anyway, and I was shocked to learn that the misdiagnosis of breast cancer in young women was very common. Intrigued, I ordered the major reference source, eager to learn more.

A few weeks later, the desired resource, "The Delayed Diagnosis of Symptomatic Breast Cancer" by Dr. Kenneth A. Kern from the book, The Breast: Comprehensive Management of Benign and Malignant Disease, Second Edition, arrived in the mail. Immediately, I intently read the section on breast misdiagnosis. As I studied it, I was shocked to learn that the delayed diagnosis of breast can be the result of false negative fine needle aspiration, FNA, where pathologists occasionally misinterpret the FNA. I had never thought of an error by a pathologist before. Suddenly, something clicked in my mind, and I wondered if my original 2001 FNA had been misread. Worried, I asked Isaac if he thought my pathologist, Dr. Lyon, could have erred. However, he did not think that Dr. Lyon would have made a mistake, commenting that she had an impeccable record. Nonetheless, he agreed that my attorney should have the slides re-read. Consequently, Isaac signed the slides out and brought them to our attorney meeting in March.

At this meeting, I was very impressed with Attorney Rich. He was a warm medium-built man that was dressed in a mint dark suit. He had serious, bright blue eyes that sparkled with energy as he rattled, "Hello,

Robin and Dr. Gray. It is nice to meet you and work with people that are bright and educated. I'm happy to let you both know that I may not have been the smartest person in my graduating class, but I have twenty solid years of successful experience in my field. I have reviewed the medical records, and it appears you have a good case against Dr. Loh. He negligently failed to diagnose you, Robin , and as a result, you had a bad outcome with a worse prognosis," stated the attorney with a hungry grin.

"That's right Mr. Rich," I cried. "Dr. Loh certainly deserves this lawsuit if he couldn't properly diagnose cancer after five office visits. However, I also recently read that if not all the negligent doctors in a suit are sued prior to their statute of limitations, then the ones sued can exonerate themselves. Further, I have also recently read that pathology-reading errors are rare but can occur. So I think we ought to have my 2001 fine needle aspiration pathology slides re-read by a pathologist, just in case there was a mistake."

"Here are Robin 's initial 2001 breast fine needle aspiration slides that I recently signed out from Dr. Lyon's pathology lab," stated Isaac. "Please have a good pathologist recheck these slides for error. Of course, I doubt that Dr. Lyon would have made a mistake, but I guess we better check her out to cover our bridges."

"Thanks, I'll have these slides re-read by a pathologist as soon as possible," replied Attorney Rich. "We'll file the lawsuit against Dr. Loh soon."

"Well, what about the radiologist in this case. Should he be sued too?" I inquired.

Then Isaac said, "Regardless of the mammography findings, the radiologist made the ultimate appropriate surgical referral. Therefore, I really don't see how he could be liable for negligence. I don't want to look sue happy. I do need to live in this community."

"I don't believe in 'shot-gunning' either, Dr. Gray," piped up Attorney Rich. "The goal is to litigate against the physicians who are truly liable. Otherwise, a lot time and money will be wasted for nothing. By the way, I know how hard it is to be diagnosed with cancer. A very close family member of mine is a cancer survivor," added the attorney consolingly. "You might say that I somewhat understand how you folks must feel, and I'll do my best to take care of your case."

"Thanks, it was good to meet you, and I'm glad we finally have a good lawyer," I announced with a friendly smile as we departed.

As the spring of 2003 rolled in, Isaac and I traveled back to the Memorial Sloan-Kettering Cancer Center again so I could complete my reconstruction surgery. In this surgery, my temporary tissue expander implant was removed and a new implant was inserted. The surgery went painfully well and delivered me with a busting new figure, making me feel a lot more feminine.

With my breast cancer surgeries and treatments finally over, I celebrated life by spending time with my family. In June of 2003, we vacationed at my hometown in Baltimore, Maryland, to be with parents and siblings. While we were there, we also enjoyed some time with our children at the nearby Hershey Park. In moments of joy with my kids, I almost forgot about my cancer nightmare and hoped, in time, it would become a very faded distant memory.

Chapter Learning Tips

The following suggestions may be helpful to you to those who are diagnosed with breast cancer.

1. Seek out second opinions from doctor sub-specialty areas (medical oncology, plastic surgery, breast surgeon, radiation oncologist, and so on) that will be involved in your cancer treatment plan.

2. Read about your particular breast cancer sub-type and appropriate treatments.

3. Obtain online support through groups like breastcancer.org, youngsurvival.org, her2support.org and so on.

4. Consider outside help with meals and cleaning.

Chapter 5

Discovery of More Doctor Errors

We don't want to send a panic among everybody that their biopsies are wrong," says pathologist Jonathan Epstein, M.D. But there's a sizable minority, maybe 2-3 percent, who have a wrong diagnosis or who could have a more accurate diagnosis.

_Hopkins Medical News, Winter 2001

The early part of the summer in 2003 was peaceful with clear skies at the mountain behind my home. However, when July arrived, a dark gray cloud hovered over, bringing with it torrential continuous rains, flooding my backyard and lower level of our house.

I felt disappointed that God was allowing more challenges in my life and wondered if this unusual rainstorm was some kind of bad foreshadowing for something yet to occur in my life. Whatever it meant, it certainly reminded me of my recent bad luck with cancer. The flood made a mess of the inside and outside of our home, just like my delayed breast cancer diagnosis had made a mess of my internal and external body. However, unlike my body, the land and home was repairable with enough money.

Indeed, the estimate for flood repairs was expensive, amounting to over 20,000 dollars. Of course, our homeowner's insurance would not cover flood damages, so we took a fat second mortgage on our home, which only added to our enormous New York City cancer loans from the prior year.

During my endless flood clean up, I threw out many material possessions, but it did not bother me-- only my cancer diagnosis plagued my mind. As I thought about it, I was perplexed how cancer ended up in my lymph node since I only had a precancerous lump, which normally does not invade into the lymph nodes. I also wondered if some unidentified areas of invasive breast cancer had existed in my removed breast lumpectomy mass and had been missed in pathology analysis.

Annoyed with my question, I decided that I wanted a third medical opinion on my 2002 lumpectomy slides by an outstanding expert. Therefore, I called the office of a leading DCIS breast pathologist, Dr. Lagios, who I had learned of on the Internet to see if he could help me. Fortunately, his secretary told me that Dr. Lagios could render another opinion on my slides and that I should mail them to him.

Therefore, I drove to the local Cedar's Hospital pathology department, with my son, Jay, to authorize my lumpectomy pathology slides to be mailed to Dr. Lagios. When I arrived at the lab, I happened to meet a kind middle-aged male doctor with dark hair who said, "Hi, my name is Dr. Neuron. What can I do for you?"

"Hi my name is Robin Gray. I'm Dr. Gray's wife and this is my youngest son, Jay. I hope we're not disturbing you, but I have some questions about my lumpectomy slides. Furthermore, I'd like to mail my slides out for a third pathology opinion."

"Why do you desire a third opinion, dear?"

"Well, I don't understand how I could have only a precancerous mass, DCIS, and have positive micro-invasion into my regional lymph nodes."

"I see. Why don't we look at your slides together here in the binocular microscope?"

"Sure that sounds like a great idea. Maybe I'm just too obsessed with my lumpectomy pathology report, but Dr. Loh did misdiagnose my breast lump for seventeen-months. As a result, I find that it's hard for me to trust things anymore."

"Yes, I understand, and I feel for you and Dr. Gray. If you were my wife, I'd be extremely upset about your delayed cancer diagnosis. It's not good that your cancer spread into your lymph nodes. Furthermore, I see that your cancer was high-grade, which is a very poor prognostic feature. High-grade tumors are very aggressive and have a high mitotic rate of growth where cancer can spread faster than low-grade tumors."

"I've read about that recently, but at least I had intravenous CMF chemotherapy for six months and a mastectomy, so I've done everything possible to prevent a recurrence. Still, my outcome would have been much better, if Dr. Loh had diagnosed me correctly. His error is very upsetting, and I've filed a medical malpractice lawsuit against him," I angrily announced.

"Oh, I see. You know, in cases like this, you must look into everything, and if you had a mammogram, you would want to have it checked at a major medical center for accuracy," Dr. Neuron assured.

"Hmm, I see."

Well, if you had any other diagnostic tests, you would want them checked out too. Did you have a biopsy?" asked Dr. Neuron with his eyebrows raised.

"Yes, I had a fine needle aspiration biopsy done in 2001."

"Oh, you did," nodded Dr. Neuron. "Well, dear, then you should have the fine needle aspiration slides reviewed by an out-of-town 'breast' pathologist to check its accuracy."

"Well, my lawyer has my 2001 fine needle aspiration biopsy slides in his possession. He assured me that he was going to have them appropriately checked."

"Oh, I see."

"Dr. Neuron, the reason I wanted to speak to you is that I'm confused as to why my lymph node contained cancer. You see, I only had a precancerous breast lump, which doesn't normally invade into the lymph nodes. However, mine oddly did. I wonder if I really did have a small invasive cancer that was somehow missed and not cut into breast slides for pathology evaluation."

"Uh-huh, that's always possible, as we don't assess the entire lumpectomy specimen because that would be impossible. However, extremely thin slices; only microns large, from various sections of the specimen are made to make sure the slides are as representative as possible."

"Well, I had a very large tumor, Dr. Neuron, and an invasive cancer could have been missed. I just hope that my lumpectomy breast slides were cut in the area where my eight by five-millimeter mammography calcification was. Personally, I would think that tiny calcification is the place where an invasive cancer would most likely be found in my large, five to seven centimeter, lumpectomy specimen."

"Really, let's look at your slides together through this double-headed microscope for two people. I notice the areas of high-grade comedo DCIS on these numerous slides. Also, I see many tiny calcifications in all your slides. Do you see that?"

"I'm not sure because I'm not a pathologist."

"Let me get a book on breast pathology to show you what calcifications look like." As he was gone, I noticed Dr. Lyon's plagues of training from various respected hospitals on the wall, which only made me feel more secure with my initial fine needle aspiration results, knowing she had read my slides.

Finally, Dr. Neuron came back blurting, "Robin, here's the book I was looking for." Then he opened it up and pointed at a photograph of DCIS with micro-calcifications, lecturing, "You see what micro-calcifications look like now and there are calcifications throughout all your slides, not just the slides with the questionable micro-invasion."

"Yes, what you are saying about scattered calcifications may be true on a microscopic level. However, I'm specifically interested in the single mammography calcification I had, which is much bigger than the microscopic calcifications on these slides. One of my breast pathology slides must correlate with the mammography calcification found on my final mammogram. I'd like to have that slide reviewed because if I had an invasive cancer, I would think that slide would show it."

"I don't know about that, Robin. The only area I see suspicious for invasive cancer is on the slide with questionable micro-invasion. However, I believe the questionable micro-invasion is slicing artifact and not real micro-invasion," announced Dr. Neuron with assurance. "You see, when pathology slides are prepared, we make thin tumor slices where the cutting can cause tiny areas of pseudo-invasion, which is due to the slicing and not real invasion. I believe that is what is present in your pathology. Therefore, I'd have to agree with the diagnosis of high-grade comedo DCIS with questionable micro-invasion. As I understand it, the second opinion on your lumpectomy from New York City Pathology didn't identify invasive breast cancer."

"Correct, Dr. Neuron, they only reported precancerous areas and some areas suspicious for micro-invasion, so I don't understand how cancer cells escaped the ducts and ended up in the regional lymph nodes."

"Again, there's always a small potential to miss an invasive cancer, but numerous slides are normally made to help decrease the chances of missing something important. Then we keep a small tissue block for the patient, but the bulk of the tumor is discarded after a few weeks."

"Great," I replied in frustration, knowing that my tossed tumor may have contained a hidden invasive breast cancer.

"Well, I see you are upset, Robin. However, I notice that your surgeon made just over twenty-five slides. This is more than the normal and commendable. You were also treated with chemotherapy, which should help prevent any potential cancer relapse. I wish you the very best."

ruuntss оп

"Thanks for your help and your generous time, Dr. Neuron. I guess I won't be sending these slides out after all. I feel comfortable with your verbal pathology analysis on my lumpectomy slides."

As soon as Jay and I got home, I replayed the Dr. Neuron's visit in my mind. When I got to the part of him telling me to double check mammography and pathology reports, in a case of litigation, I stopped dead in my thoughts. Immediately, I wondered what Attorney Rich's pathologist had found on the review of my 2001 initial breast fine needle aspiration slides, and I wondered why I had not heard about the review. Therefore, I dialed my lawyer.

"Hello, Attorney Rich. You know, I never heard from you regarding the pathology review on my 2001 fine needle aspiration breast pathology slides."

"Hi, Robin, everything was fine. No cancer was found on your slides."

"Really? Well, I would like to have written documentation of that report."

"Robin, I don't have a report. I had a neuropathologist, who I know well, examine the slides. To keep cost down, he didn't issue a formal report. Anyway, I thought this case was about Dr. Loh and not the pathologist."

"Yes, this case is about Dr. Loh, and I don't want him off the hook. However, I thought we had to check all possibilities out for physician error," I cried.

"Yes, and my associate pathologist didn't find cancer on your breast slides, and I think you can trust his opinion," Attorney Rich assured.

"Maybe you're right, but I think a 'breast' pathologist should have read those slides. Anyway, let me think about the way you handled the pathology review, and I'll speak to you soon," I replied with an unsettled mind.

When I got off the phone, I was disturbed because I desperately wanted written documentation on my 2001 fine needle aspiration slides. Furthermore, I did not think a neurological pathologist could adequately evaluate my breast slides, and I wanted another pathology review. Furthermore, I wanted it as fast as possible, as I realized that the statute of limitations for me litigating against Dr. Lyon was expiring within two weeks.

When Isaac got home that night, I told him the situation. He was also extremely annoyed that a neurological pathologist reviewed my breast slides. He suggested that we play it cautious and get the slides assessed again by a breast or general pathologist who would also issue us documentation of the pathology review.

Consequently, I immediately called my lawyer, requesting him to mail me my pathology slides. That way, I would have them to mail out for another more appropriate pathology review. At the same time my husband made some phone calls and found a pathologist, Dr. Wright, who agreed to analyze my 2001 fine needle aspiration biopsy slides as soon as possible. Of course, we were thankful for Dr. Wright's help, but we also had a gut feeling that his review would be consistent with Dr. Lyon's initial report.

Surprisingly, about ten days later, I received a phone call from Isaac early in the morning. He asked if I was sitting down in a very serious tone, and I knew something was wrong.

"Robin, I just got a very interesting call from Dr. Wright. He said that he found cancerous, suspicious cells in your March 2001 fine needle aspiration slides, which Dr. Lyon had read as benign. In addition, he said that three other pathologists from his lab looked at the slides, independently without his interpretation, and they all came up with the same suspicious diagnosis. Apparently, the slides were a bit cloudy, but everyone still identified a problem. Dr. Lyon did put in her report that the slides were adequate for evaluation, so she can't claim that she couldn't read the slides. Amazingly, it looks like Dr. Loh is not the only guilty party. Can you believe it? I'm shocked!"

"Oh my, I cried with utter surprise."

"I know you're upset, Robin. Do you want me to come home?"

"No, I'll be okay, Isaac," I stated. "You've got work to do, and I need to call my lawyer. At least I know the truth now about her too! Thanks."

When I got off the phone, I cried like a baby and felt devastated over all of the by not having the slides read by the appropriate person, and I was beginning to wonder whom I could trust.

Even so, I had to trust my attorney now with only forty-eight hours to file a summons and complaint on Dr. Lyon. Therefore, I immediately called him with the news, stating, "Hi Steven, guess what I just found out? My initial breast pathology slides were misread by Dr. Lyon."

"What? Are you sure?" he gasped in dismay.

"I'm sure the fine needle aspiration slides were misread. Four different pathologists all agreed that the slides were highly suspicious for cancer and that another biopsy should have been recommended."

"I feel terrible that my pathologist friend didn't catch this mistake. I'm so very sorry," Attorney Rich stated with great remorse in his voice.

"You better file a summons and complaint on Dr. Lyon. Her two-and-a-half year statute of limitation runs out in forty-eight hours. If she gets off the hook, so will Dr. Loh, and our case will be completely gone!"

"Don't worry. I'll get the summons and complaint out to the courthouse in your town immediately. She'll be served her papers sometime after that," assured Attorney Rich.

"Please make sure you get those documents out promptly. I can't afford to lose this case against them," I begged.

"Right, we've got to move on this. Look, I want you to know that there is no way that I'm letting Dr. Loh off the hook, either, even with this initial pathology error. A negative fine needle aspiration was meaningless with a persistent and enlarging breast lump."

"You're right, Steven, Dr. Loh is still guilty. Just please make the deadline," I begged.

After my conversation with my attorney, I felt enraged with Dr. Lyon. I could not believe her error with all the excellent training and experience she had. Furthermore, I had a good hunch she knew of her error when I spoke to her, months earlier, about my pathology slides and misdiagnosis. Of course, why should she tell me about her pathology reading error?

Furious, I gave her a call at her office. Of course, when I told her that I knew she misread my slides, she denied her error and told me she read them correctly. Frustrated, I informed her that she could defend herself in legal deposition, and then I hung up the phone in disgust.

After the phone call, I decided not only would I certainly sue Dr. Lyon, but also I would follow and record every detail of the lawsuit carefully, especially after my attorney's screw-up too. Consequently, I phoned Dr. Wright for a written copy of my fine needle aspiration biopsy report, which contradicted Dr. Lyon's report. However, to my surprise, Dr. Wright did not want to give me the report, stating that he knew Dr. Lyon and Dr. Loh and he did not want to get involved with my litigation case. Then Dr. Wright suggested that my attorney find a new pathologist to blow the whistle on Dr. Lyon's error.

Undeterred, I phoned one of the other pathologists in Dr. Wright's office who had also reviewed my slides and found them to be cancerous. Fortunately, this pathologist very kindly agreed to mail me her report on my fine needle aspiration slides. I certainly was impressed with the honesty and assistance of this physician, who I did not even know. This individual greatly helped to somewhat restore my faith in doctors.

Still, following my physician-related errors and attorney errors, I developed a paranoid feeling of mistrust with professionals, particularly with physicians. In fact, I began to question all my medical care.

I worried if my gynecology oncologist, Dr. Dubester, who I had recently seen for an ovarian mass, was correct in diagnosing me with a benign cyst. I worried that the ovarian cyst was actually cancer so much that I had it surgically removed. Fortunately, the ovarian cyst pathology was benign via three separate pathology opinions.

While I was recovering from the ovarian surgery, I also began to question my DCIS (precancerous) pathology diagnosis on my lumpectomy slides again. I figured if Dr. Lyon had made a mistake on my 2001 fine needle aspiration slides, then pathology errors were also possible on my 2002 lumpectomy slides.

Curiously, I checked the credentials of the pathologist, Dr. Daniels, who reviewed my 2002 lumpectomy pathology slides at the New York City Pathology Group. I was shocked to learn that this pathologist was an anatomical pathologist and not a breast pathologist. Enraged over my finding, I immediately mailed my lumpectomy slides out to the New York City Pathology Group and specifically requested that a breast pathologist render yet another opinion on my lumpectomy slides.

About two weeks later, I was peacefully playing with my youngest son, Jay, when I suddenly got a phone call from the breast pathologist from the New York City Pathology Group .

"Hello, this is Dr. Moon from the New York City Pathology Group. I've been trying to reach you about your breast lumpectomy slides. I discovered that you had more than just a precancerous mass or DCIS. You also had a small invasive cancer on your lumpectomy slides. Furthermore, the invasive cancer was both estrogen and progesterone negative and positive for HER2, an aggressive poor prognostic marker. I'm very sorry to have to inform you of this. I've consulted with Dr. Daniels, who did the initial pathology reading, and he has amended his report to include this new invasive cancer discovery."

"Oh my God!" I gasped with horror. "How could he make such an error? I only had CMF chemotherapy and probably should have had the more aggressive AC chemotherapy with this aggressive cancer subtype.

How in the world could Dr. Daniels from your esteemed pathology group have missed this invasive cancer? This is the fourth breast pathology error I've encountered. What a medical error nightmare! First, I had a seventeen-month delayed diagnosis of breast cancer partly due to my local pathologist, Dr. Lyon, misreading my breast fine needle aspiration slides. Now, I find that two local pathologists and your larger center misread my surgical lumpectomy slides. What are the odds of that happening? I recently read that pathology errors account for only 1 percent of breast cancer misdiagnosis, but I guess not in my case."

"Mrs. Gray, I'm so sorry this is happening to you."

"Dr. Moon, why did your center ever send breast slides to an anatomical pathologist to begin with and not a breast pathologist?"

"We only have one breast pathologist here, and sometimes we get so busy that we can't read all of the breast specimens. When that occurs, the slides go to another specialty pathologist who isn't busy. All of our pathologists are trained to cross read other specialty slides."

"That certainly is a dangerous policy from an acclaimed cancer pathology group. What type of HER2 testing did you perform, as you say I'm HER2 positive? I'll need to know in case I need more chemotherapy treatment or Herceptin."

"There wasn't enough tissue to do the fluorescence in situ hybridization test or FISH test, which is the more accurate one to assess the amount of over expression of HER2. I used the immunohistochemistry test or IHC test on your breast cancer tissue block. But I got the highest level of over-expression possible, which is +3. I do a lot of the IHC testing, and I definitely feel your breast cancer would have tested positive for the more accurate FISH test as well."

"Great, I'm strongly positive for HER2, which is not good. Now I'm going to have to see my oncologist to see what kind of further cancer treatment I may need."

"Mrs. Gray, I'm very sorry about this late diagnosis. If there is anything further I can do for you, please call me personally at my office."

"Thank you for finding the error and for being candid in reporting it to me. I appreciate it."

When I got off the phone, I just shook with fear, and tears ran down my face. I felt defeated over, yet, another medical mistake. Furthermore, I was shaken that my invasive cancer had worse biological markers, estrogen negative and HER2 positive, which indicated that my breast cancer was more aggressive.

As I worried about everything with tears in my eyes, I made a phone call to my local general oncologist and updated him on the new discovery. He reassured me that I did have chemotherapy and not to worry.

Still, after I hung up the phone, I was filled with anxiety and desired another oncology opinion on my new findings. Therefore, I called my oncologist from Memorial Sloan-Kettering and explained the situation. However, she reassured me also that I had chemotherapy and required no further treatment.

Fearful with previous physician errors, I was still worried, desiring, yet, another expert oncology opinion. Therefore, I made an appointment with an esteemed oncologist, Dr. Leroy Parker, from the Dana Faber

Cancer Center in Boston, Massachusetts. I also forwarded my lumpectomy breast slides to the Dana Faber Cancer Center for a fifth opinion.

Finally, after a long Christmas holiday spent worrying about my medical mishaps, I ended up at Dr. Parker's Boston office in early January 2004. To my relief, Dr. Parker agreed with the previous oncologists and informed me that no further treatment would be recommended at such a late date. He also assured me that my prognosis was excellent after my various medical treatments, stating that it would be difficult to prove that CMF was less effective than the more aggressive AC chemotherapy for HER2 positive breast cancer. Finally, with his opinions, I felt that no more treatments were needed.

Still, I was upset that the New York City Pathology Group had made such a big pathology error, so I wrote them a letter where I complained about their pathology errors. Much to our surprise, they did acknowledge my complaint and apologized.

As spring arrived, I developed intense headaches, and I worried if it could be a brain metastasis, as I read that hormonal negative HER2 positive breast cancer had an affinity to spread into the central nervous system. Consequently, I saw a neurologist who scheduled a Magnetic Resonance Imaging (MRI) of my brain. Fortunately, nothing unusual was found, and a few weeks later the headaches mysteriously vanished.

I was very thankful that my head pain subsided and that my MRI was fine, but at the same time, I was angry that I had to worry about such things as brain metastasis. I wanted to talk to others in the same boat as me and express some of my anxieties and anger issues. I was fortunate to find the Young Survival Coalition (YSC) website, which is a support group for young breast cancer survivors.

As I began to express my concerns on the YSC discussion boards, I surprisingly found someone else who was supportive of me. Her husband was also a physician and her breast lump was misdiagnosed for fifteen months, part of the time, when she was pregnant. Of course, getting to know her made me feel better about my misdiagnosis, realizing I was not alone. She also informed me that she dealt with her misdiagnosis by not dealing with the 'whys and what ifs.'

I viewed this new friend as strong-minded and only wished to be as mighty in acceptance as her. However, I just seemed powerless and could not shake my anger with the physicians who misdiagnosed me. Sadly, sometimes I was even mad at my husband for referring me to such incompetent physicians. Other times, I was mad at myself for having trusted my physicians. My anger was unpleasant; however, at least it distracted from my worse emotion, fear of a cancer relapse.

However, fear did eventually rear its ugly head as summer approached when I was on the YSC discussion board website. It seemed like many of the other young women with HER2 positive breast cancer on the discussion board had more aggressively treatments than I had. They had stronger chemotherapy with a new adjuvant anti-HER2 treatment called Herceptin. Naturally, I worried if I had been under-treated, not having Herceptin, especially since I had a weaker chemotherapy regimen than most. As my world of anxiety grew, I started to feel overwhelmed with my breast cancer nightmare and the events of the proceeding two years...

I missed the old carefree Robin. I worried continuously about whether I should have had Herceptin, even though it had not been recommended by my many oncologists. Furthermore, the misdiagnosis and life-saving poison of chemotherapy had changed me. I suffered restless nights and was totally out of my self with changes and medical problems.

I prayed for normalcy and health to come back to me. However, nothing happened, and I felt like pieces of me were scattered about. I tried to pick them up, but too much was broken.

Within the broken pieces about me, I saw the reflection of what had gone so wrong. It was the neglect of doctors. They left a hollow vacuum in my chest, and it sucked in my mind, robbing me of peace.

It seemed like the only thing that was left in my head were feelings of humiliation, betrayal, fear, and loss. However, the feeling of loss haunted me the most, and it pushed me into a cold, dark hole, depriving me of sleep for several nights. I prayed feverishly for God to give me peace and rest; however, sleep evaded me. Therefore, in despair and in physical pain from exhaustion, I took numerous sleeping medications to resolve my insomnia, but it failed to help me. Finally, I was treated for severe depression and given some anti-depressants, stronger sleep aids, and some therapeutic counseling.

Fortunately, the psychological treatments lifted my sadness, sense of loss, and insomnia, propelling me to get on with my life in a new and positive light. I made a self-commitment to focus on the good in my life and not to focus on the ills of the past.

In fact, I thought that I would even drop the lawsuits in order to put my medical disaster behind me. I may have dropped the case, too; however, my husband and his office physician peers encouraged me to not give up and to make Dr. Loh and Dr. Lyon accountable for their negligent errors so others would not suffer from their careless mistakes.

Chapter Learning Tips

The following list of suggestions may help those who were misdiagnosed, prior to reading this book:

1. Prior to beginning a lawsuit, decide whether you wish to talk to your physician(s) about the medical error(s) that you think occurred. You may want to take someone with you to help record the events.
2. Obtain your medical records and examine them for errors.
3. Obtain second opinions on reports such as mammograms, ultrasounds, and breast biopsies to see if they agree with the initial reports, noting doctor errors.
4. Make a list of the doctor errors and determine if your case meets the three criteria a for a medical malpractice lawsuit discussed at the beginning of chapter six.
5. Find out the statue of limitations or legal time frame where you have to sue your physician(s) and make sure you start a malpractice suit within this period, if you decide to sue.
6. Note the stage of cancer you have and if you can litigate. Unfortunately, in some states, you must have a stage three cancer or higher to litigate.

7. If you decide to litigate, make a historical record of the events of your misdiagnosis, including dates of doctor visits, tests, and so on.

8. Select a malpractice attorney that is experienced in breast litigation and has a positive record in settlements.

Chapter 6

Lawsuits and Depositions

Some medical practitioners apparently feel that they should have immunity from any punishment for their malpractice. Not only do they feel that their actions should not subject them to punishment, but they will go to almost any length to prevent being exposed.

_ Lethal Medicine, 1993

Now that I was recovering from anxiety and depression, I decided to take things easy for a while. I spent several days on the back porch of my home, rocking in a chair overlooking the mountain where I lived while I watched my boys play in the backyard. I was glad to be with my kids and hoped that I could keep my troubles behind me.

However, a few weeks into my recovery, my upsetting cancer misdiagnosis whirled into my mind when my lawyer phoned. He wanted me to meet him this time at his big city office, two hours away, rather than in the small upstate New York town that I lived in, so we could discuss the medical malpractice deposition, which was coming up soon. Emotionally, I still felt shaky, but I agreed to the meeting, wanting to prove to everyone that I could handle things.

The night before the meeting, I glanced at my old notes and outline that cited Dr. Loh and Dr. Lyon's medical malpractice. As I read the following summary outline, it was quite apparent that the doctors filled the three criteria necessary for medical malpractice: (1) the existence of a duty imposed by law; (2) a breach of that duty; and (3) damage caused by the breach of duty.

Medical Malpractice Summary

A. Evidence of Physician Negligence

1. Dr. Loh- The following errors by my general surgeon formed the central argument for his negligence:

- Failure to explain to me the benefit of an immediate breast biopsy on the first visit or perform a biopsy, which would have given me the best opportunity for early diagnosis and revealed the histological make-up of my breast lump. (See postscript, on page 99, to see why a breast biopsy is vital. to give early diagnosis.)

- Erroneously told me that my breast lump was not suspicious for cancer on the first visit when Dr. Covington documented it as 'suspicious' and when it ultimately did prove cancerous.

- In the first few visits, not only neglected to do the necessary breast biopsy, but falsely diagnosed my lump as benign fibrocystic condition when it was really cancerous.

- Never did a breast biopsy until four months later, at my third visit. Even then, the doctor failed to tell me about the more accurate core or excisional biopsy and only did a fine needle aspiration biopsy. (See postscript which explains the risk of fine needle aspiration biopsy and how other biopsy types are more reliable.)

- Failure to acknowledge a suspicious clinical breast exam, as evidenced by positive brown nipple drainage and persistent growth of lump over time. (See postscripts for warnings on brown nipple drainage and persistent growth of a breast lump.)

- Failure to do prompt follow-up appointment following the fine needle aspiration in order to see if lump had resolved or persisted. (See postscripts to see why a persistent lump must NOT be ignored but must be removed.)

- At the ten-month follow-up appointment, failure to excise persistent and enlarging mass. (See postscript which explains why a persistent lump demands removal.)

2. Dr. Lyon- Failure to diagnose breast fine needle aspiration slides accurately, erroneously making a benign fibrocystic diagnosis on cloudy slides that were not even adequate for evaluation.

B. Patient Damages Due To Misdiagnosis

1. A mastectomy rather than lumpectomy - lost breast due to large size of DCIS.

2. An additional excisional surgery after my mastectomy due to extensive growth of my DCIS outside the boundaries of a normal mastectomy.

3. Presence of cancer in the lymph node due to the fact that my untreated DCIS invaded.

- Necessity of intravenous chemotherapy for a positive lymph node.
- Sentinel node axillary dissection surgery, which is only done when DCIS is large, as mine was due to my delayed cancer diagnosis.
- Increased cancer stage with decrease in disease free survival due to cancer spread into my lymph node.

4. Chronic pain of right arm due to sentinel node dissection, a surgery which could have been prevented with early diagnosis.

5. Emotional pain and distress due to all the above and constant reminder of events due to the surgical scars, loss of breast, and chemotherapy induced hormonal deprivation.

6. Multiple medical bills amounting to thousands of dollars that my health insurance would not pay.

It was depressing to read my doctors' errors, so I did not really dwell on the above outline long. Besides the details of the misdiagnosis were fresh in my mind anyway, like a mint coin, so I went to bed.

The following day, Isaac and I took off for the long trip to see my attorney. When we finally got there, we were warmly greeted by Mr. Rich, as he welcomed us to his big fancy office, which was decorated with fine furniture, screaming he had won a number of lawsuits. I felt certainly felt impressed, hoping he would settle my case, too.

Then my attorney rambled on for a while, informing us that the deposition would not be bad, and the only thing I had to do was tell the truth as simply as possible. Furthermore, he announced that my case might settle soon. Upon hearing that, I informed my attorney that I would give my negligent doctors the olive branch of forgiveness if they would expediently end the case with a payment and confession.

However, the following day at deposition, when Isaac, my attorney, and I met with the opposing attorneys, there was nothing at all amicable or peaceful in the air. The negligent physicians' attorneys stared at me like a couple of hungry wolves as my stomach churned with nervous spasms. Then, one at a time, they began firing endless questions, concerning dates and details of various physicians that I had seen me in the past ten years. I was very surprised and appalled that they had obviously delved into my very distant medical records, prior to my misdiagnosis.

Finally, they got in to the misdiagnosis and asked me a ton of questions. They bombarded me with so many inquiries that I eventually got a sore throat from talking so much, and I felt mentally exhausted near the end of my three-hour long interrogation.

When it was all over, I was amazed at what they put me through when the doctors were obviously in error; not the patient. At least, the dirty ordeal was over, and I felt as if I had done a good job answering the questions fully, honestly, and to the best of my ability.

About a week after my deposition, my attorney deposed and questioned Dr. Loh and Dr. Lyon. I was expecting the same honesty that I had shelled out with their admission and confession of guilt. However, when my attorney finished questioning them, he immediately called me with a frustrating update.

"Robin, I just deposed Dr. Loh and Dr. Lyon, and I have bad news. Neither of them admitted guilt!"

"How can they have the audacity to deny wrong doing?" I screamed in dismay.

"I know it gets me too. First off, I nearly fell off my chair when Dr. Lyon denied seeing cancer on your slides after she rechecked them in 2003, after your misdiagnosis."

"Steven, I can't believe she lied under oath!"

"I know, me too. Dr. Lyon dressed finely and looked like a nice woman at first, but when she didn't come forth with the truth, I changed my opinion of her character. I can't believe she is trying to deny the obvious. She's hiding a lot. She even refused to tell me what her partner saw when they viewed the slides. Don't you worry, though. I'm going to seek the judge out to try to depose Dr. Lyon's partners."

"Good, and what about Dr. Loh? What did he say?"

"I'm not as surprised, but I am sorry to say that Dr. Loh, also, refused to admit guilt. I could tell he was lying throughout his entire deposition," wined Attorney Rich depressingly.

"That stinks," I cried.

"Don't worry, we're going after these people, they're not going to get away with anything."

"That's right, Steven, those people don't know who they are dealing with and how tough and tenacious we are."

"Right, if they want to drag this to court, then we're prepared to go there to win this case. In fact, maybe I would like it that way."

"I'm glad you're not afraid of them, Steven. I'm with you 100 percent. Thanks for the update."

When I got off the phone, Isaac and I felt devastated by his colleagues' lies, indifferent stonewalling, and betrayal. At least their lying did not send me off the deep end this time, as luckily, my Zoloft seemed to be working well.

As the autumn pressed on, I grew more and more emotionally optimistic. However, the misdiagnosis was still spinning in the back of my mind. I often thought how ironic it was that the first "her too" discovery, concerning Dr. Lyon's error, led to the "HER2" invasive breast cancer discovery error. Cognizant of my extraordinary medical mishaps, I feverishly commenced the writing of my story. I was determined to ventilate my frustrations and turn my darkest days into brighter ones via helping others.

At the end of November, my lawyer called to let me know that he had appeared before the upstate New York judge appointed to my case. He asked the judge if she would demand Dr. Lyon's partners to divulge their 2003 pathology findings on my fine needle aspiration slides. My lawyer thought Dr. Lyon's partners should discuss the truth of their findings, which he felt would convict Dr. Lyon clearly and encourage her to settle before trail.

Stirred by my lawyer appearing before the judge in November, I thought it was time for me to read the depositions from the prior summer that I had never seen. Therefore, I called my attorney for the deposition transcripts.

A few days later, I got them in the mail. As I read them over, I was astonished to see that my personal deposition was thick at 142 pages long, but the depositions of the physicians were only 41-51 pages long each. I thought it was ironic and outrageous that I had been questioned much more extensively than my negligent physicians.

Still, I was calm as I started to read the transcripts. I did not think I would learn anything new or upsetting from the transcripts since my lawyer had given me a summary of the transcripts several months earlier. However, I was horrified as I read Dr. Loh's transcript and his litany of twisted truths. In astonishment, I ran for my husband.

"Isaac, I just read Dr. Loh's deposition. I can't believe he not only denied his errors, but he blamed me for the misdiagnosis!" I cried.

"What exactly did he say in deposition?" demanded Isaac.

"He stated that the lump didn't stand out as suspicious, was not a 'progressive thing, growing over time and that it only was 'beginning cancer' when he removed it at the time of the lumpectomy," I announced with anger.

"That's ridiculous!" screamed Isaac. "That lump was documented by Dr. Covington as only a tiny mass back in November of 2000. However, by the time Dr. Loh removed it in 2002, it was two to three inches large! So how can Dr. Loh deny your cancer's growth?

"Right, how can he deny it when he even documented my lump as bigger in the four-month follow-up medical note? Plus, Dr. Loh and the nurse documented, at the ten-month follow-up, that I reported that the lump was larger."

"Well, then he can't deny that it was growing," yelled Isaac.

"Yes, but he did," I snapped in frustration. "In deposition, he stated that even though I (the patient) felt the lump was larger at the ten-month follow up visit, he didn't do a repeat biopsy because he didn't think the lump was bigger. However, he didn't tell me, at that visit, that he didn't agree with my report of an enlarging lump. He only reassured me that the lump was fibrocystic and could enlarge without harm."

"He knows that lump was enlarging. He just lied in deposition to protect his butt," cried Isaac.

"Your right, hon. Anyway, he should have kept a record of the lump's growth if he was assessing something that was possibly cancerous."

"You're right, Robin."

"He makes me sick in the deposition with all his lies. What a coward. He claimed that he only gave me a '95 percent' certainty that I had a benign lump. What a crock, I certainly wouldn't have ignored a 5 percent risk of cancer if I had known about such a risk. I would have demanded that the lump come out," I yelled. "He always told me that my lump was not suspicious for cancer."

"Right," added Isaac. "Nor did he tell me that your lump was suspicious for cancer."

"Right, but in the deposition, Dr. Loh stated that he always only gave the '95 percent' certain it is a benign process' script to all his breast patients. Well, he never gave me the script," I snapped.

"The whole 95 percent premise doesn't even make sense," argued Isaac. "It's outrageous that Dr. Loh would be satisfied with a 95 percent certain diagnosis when there was a 5 percent or more risk of cancer."

"Right, his premise doesn't make sense. Anyway, he assured me that my lump was not suspicious for cancer, but he cowardly did not admit that in his deposition. Plus, he outrageously blamed me for his errors. Look, here in the deposition transcripts, he stated the reason he didn't inform me of the safer core and excisional biopsy was because I didn't want a 100 percent diagnosis. How dare he use me as an excuse for not doing those safer biopsy methods! I even specifically asked him, at my third doctor visit, if the fine needle aspiration would adequately assess my breast lump, and he assured me it would, failing to tell me about the safer biopsy methods. Certainly, he failed to give me informed consent of the most accurate diagnosing options, failed to give me the most accurate core or excisional biopsy methods, and failed at his job by not diagnosing my lump correctly."

"You're right, Robin, he is one big failure, but can't admit it and shamefully blames you for his mistakes. He's despicable."

"Yes, he is. I'm shocked by his lies and by his misdiagnosis. Dr. Loh should have known how to assess breast lumps since he claimed in deposition to care for as many as 300-350 breast cases per year."

"Yes, he should have known with all of his experience over many years of practice," cried Isaac in disgust.

"Yes, he should have known what he was doing, especially with a doctor's wife. Now he's making things more difficult for us by lying about his errors," I screamed.

"His lying true character is revealed," cried Isaac. "I was willing to forgive his mistakes and move on, if he had only told the truth. He had his opportunity at deposition to come clean with his mistakes and take responsibility for them. But he didn't, he is shameful."

"He's certainly placed the surgeon's knife in our backs, severing our trust forever. What are you going to do about his false statements, Isaac?"

"Just keep it above the belt and continue with your lawsuit. Unfortunately, that's all I can do, even though I feel betrayed and violated. I definitely don't want a confrontation with Dr. Loh. In fact, when I work, I try to avoid his path the best I can because if I see him, I might lose control."

"I understand, Isaac. I thought he would have upheld the Hippocratic Oath, to do no harm to the patient. What a joke, he harms, lies about it, turns around, and blames me, the innocent patient. If he was going to blame anyone, why not Dr. Lyon for her erroneous pathology report on my fine needle aspiration?"

"He doesn't want to blame Dr. Lyon because then the doctors would be pointing fingers at each other and both would look guilty, so you're the scapegoat," argued Isaac. "By the way, where is Dr. Lyon's deposition?"

"I've got it, Isaac, and I'm reading now…Oh my, does the doctor lie? She doesn't admit that she misread my slides. Yet, she stated she recalled my case because she was surprised that only a fine needle aspiration was done for an enlarging mass. Well, then why didn't she request a more aggressive biopsy, if she felt that was inadequate?"

"I don't know," stated Isaac in disgust.

"Plus, Isaac, why didn't she take more time to look at my slides if the history of an enlarging mass appeared suspicious to her?"

"Well, because she was asleep on the darn job when she looked at your slides, Robin."

"What's wrong with your trusted colleagues, Isaac? If she had made a correct diagnosis, my delayed diagnosis would only have been four months rather than seventeen! Certainly, that would have saved me an invasive cancer, additional surgeries, chemotherapy, and a worse prognosis."

"I'm sorry that my colleagues harmed you, and then made it worse by lying and not taking responsibility for their incompetent medical care! They not only lied but have the audacity to continue practicing medicine in this small town."

"Yep, Isaac, they sure do have some nerve lying, ignoring the harm they did to me, and going on practicing as if nothing has happened. Wow, if they can lie and try to cover their errors on a doctor's wife, who is a nurse, what are they capable of doing to the unknowing average Joe? I hate to think about it and their criminal hit and run behavior, Isaac."

"Right Robin, they're not honest or trustworthy, and they have prejudiced themselves during legal deposition!"

"Yep, I hate their dishonesty and how it has further hurt our family. At the very least, couldn't they do the right thing by telling the truth and settling with us? I don't think I'm being too selfish in wanting an apology and some compensation for the suffering I've experienced due to their mistakes. They wouldn't have to pay a cent. Their malpractice insurer would pay; yet, they can't admit the truth. I'm really furious, and I'm going to hammer out a letter about these physicians to my lawyer."

When I was done writing, I thought about the range of damages from my misdiagnosis. I knew nothing could repair the physical and emotional harm that was done, not even a lawsuit payment. Full of melancholy, I longed for days past. I missed my breast, my healthy painless body, I missed my female hormones destroyed by chemotherapy, and I missed my peaceful life prior to my misdiagnosis.

I missed so much; yet, my questions of 'whys' tortured me just as much. I wondered why the doctors tried to make my wounds fester more with poison by not admitting their errors at deposition. Very baffled by their reactions, my husband and I turned to a friend and psychologist who assisted us by listening compassionately to our medical nightmare. The counseling was somewhat helpful to both of us; however, not completely.

Then I also spoke to my lawyer, Steven Rich, for his impression of why my physicians had chosen to lie at deposition. My lawyer simply explained, "Welcome to the real world where dishonest doctors make mistakes and don't admit them. Then they expect to settle the case before trail without admission of guilt or exposure of their errors."

My attorney's words were not very comforting. I was furious to think my doctors could settle without admission of guilt. I wanted them accountable for their errors and lies.

I also very much yearned to know why my physicians had made mistakes in my case. However, I realized that my negligent doctors would never give me the truth. Therefore, I began to study the medical literature to learn why my pathologist, who was highly regarded in her field, would have made such an egregious error in the interpretation of my fine needle aspiration (FNA). I learned in an article, by Karen Titus, "Breast specimens: FNA, core, more" (from *College of American Pathologists, February 2002,* page 3) that correct FNA interpretation is dependent on the pathologist's amount of experience in reading FNA biopsies. I found it interesting that if this be true, then Dr. Lyon willingly admitted, in the deposition transcripts, her lack of reading FNAs for masses by stating, 'We don't, you know, obtain that many fine needle aspirations of breast masses.'

It appeared to me that Dr. Lyon convicted herself of why the error happened. I was angry, thinking she shouldn't had been diagnosing biopsy pathology for which she felt she had inadequate experience, particularly when it involved something as serious as ruling out breast cancer in a young woman.

One day, I had the opportunity to speak with one of Dr. Lyon's former pathology partners, Dr. Cross, about Dr. Lyon's error. Of course, he did not convict his prior partner. In fact, he supported her, stating that pathology opinions could vary widely and were very subjective. Of course, I did not swallow his response well, thinking if the pathology reports were so subjective, then nobody would trust pathology reports.

In investigating the various aspects of my case, I found it an exhausting process. Once I answered one question, more arose. Mentally drained, I decided to take a long holiday Christmas break from everything.

However, as the 2005 New Year rolled in, my lawyer contacted me, and I found myself back into my lawsuit. He called to let me know that the judge would not force Dr. Lyon's pathology partners to reveal how they interpreted the slides that Dr. Lyon misread. My attorney was angry and frustrated. However, I was determined to pursue the doctors harder than ever.

Therefore, I dug a little deeper into the case by asking my attorney to send me Dr. Loh's medical requisition on my 2001 fine needle aspiration that was sent to Dr. Lyon in 2001 when she erroneously read my slides. I had actually first learned of this form when I read the physicians' recent depositions, noting that they had mentioned the requisition while questioning Dr. Loh.

When I finally received the form from my attorney, I found it interesting that Dr. Lyon missed many things on my biopsy's requisition form. First, my husband's name, Isaac Gray, was on the top of the form, in the box for person responsible for billing, above my clinical diagnosis. Yet in deposition, Dr. Lyon denied being aware that the specimen was from Isaac Gray's wife. Perhaps she just did not read the billing section. I wonder if she even read the suspicious clinical history on the requisition form, either, which stated that my 'lumps were persisting from four months prior and enlarging.' Certainly, such a suspicious history demanded a very accurate pathology reading, something that was not done by Dr. Lyon.

The requisition from Dr. Loh's records also made him look bad. On this form, Dr. Loh documented 'persistent and enlarging lumps.' Yet, in deposition, he specifically denied a lump or mass and stated that my condition was not growing.

After all my research, I certainly had no doubts that my physicians made cavalier errors in my case, which they simply failed to admit. I wondered how they managed to cope and live with themselves.

Still perplexed with my delayed cancer diagnosis in the winter of 2005, I searched the New York State Physician Profile and New York State Office of Professional Medical Conduct (OPMC) websites to see if Dr. Loh and Dr. Lyon had any malpractice lawsuit settlements listed. To my surprise, I did not see any black marks on their so-called impeccable records. At the same time, I knew not all patients litigate when errors happen or report errors to the state. Furthermore, as I read the OPMC website, I learned it does not make probationary measures on negligent physicians public where doctor re-training and monitoring occur for improved patient care.

Curious about my physicians' complete profiles, I continued to read beyond their malpractice records and learned that Dr. Lyon recorded a litany of volunteer activities and associations that she was involved with. Naturally, I wondered why she was so busy with ancillary activities if she could not even take the time to read my breast slides accurately.

As I read the Physician Profile website over again more thoroughly, I learned that physicians' complete malpractice record would not always be in the profile. I was shocked to learn that the state agency website did not fully inform the public of the physicians' medical malpractice record and that cases could settle without being listed in the physician profile record. I did not think that was very fair and wondered how else I could discover my doctors' entire malpractice record. As I thought about it, I clicked around the website for a while until I finally discovered that the way to check a physician's entire malpractice record was through the County Clerk's office where the physician practices.

Ever anxious to explore my negligent doctors' records, I immediately visited the County Clerk's office with my son, Neo. I found nothing filed with Dr. Lyon's record other than my summons and complaint. However, in Dr. Loh's record, I found that a male, Mr. X, had filed a medical malpractice claim in 2001, for of all things a breast malpractice case. Additionally, I found that the doctor had another suit against him, claiming that he had incorrectly done a tumor biopsy on a woman's arm, permanently damaging her ulnar nerve.

Particularly intrigued with my findings on Mr. X, I gave him a call about his breast misdiagnosis. According to Mr. X, Dr. Loh assessed him in 1998 for breast pain and tenderness, and Dr. Loh performed an immediate fine needle aspiration biopsy of the breast. A positive cytology cancer diagnosis was made from this aspiration, and Dr. Loh performed an immediate left mastectomy and axillary dissection. However, the pathology from this surgery revealed no cancer. According to the patient, a local pathologist misread the initial fine needle aspiration. On Jan. 10, 2001, a summons and complaint was filed by Mr. X on Dr. Loh, two local pathologists, a local hospital, and several other local medical professionals. Mr. X claimed medical negligence and injury from the unnecessary surgeries, claiming permanent scars and deformity to his body.

I was certainly amazed to hear of Mr. X's misdiagnosis, as I realized that his case appeared to be the exact mirror image of my case. Mr. X did not have a breast lump, only breast pain and tenderness. Yet, he got the immediate fine needle aspiration biopsy on his first visit to Dr. Loh that I should have gotten. Furthermore, he received the immediate surgical intervention that I so urgently needed. I could hardly believe the irony of finding out about Mr. X's case, all too late.

My new discovery was upsetting, as I wondered why Dr. Loh was not meticulous in assessing and diagnosing my breast lump when he had just been in a breast malpractice case. Surely, he would not have forgotten this embarrassing 1998 case by the time I saw him in November of 2000. In fact, how could he forget it when he was served his malpractice suit for Mr. X's case during the early phase of my misdiagnosis in 2001?

Furthermore, how could he not remember his prior bad experience with a breast fine needle aspiration, and why did he use the risky test on me? How in the world could Dr. Loh assure me of the accuracy of the fine needle aspiration when I asked him about its ability to assess my lump? He withheld, deprived, and neglected to inform me of what he well knew by current experience, stealing from me the chance for early diagnosis and treatment. His obvious cavalier approach in assessing my breast lump angered me so much that I found myself pounding on my computer keyboard, typing out his errors for my book.

As I banged on the keys, I Thought it was not very candid of Dr. Loh to inform me in the summer of 2002, during his good luck call, that he had not experienced any mistakes like mine before. In fact, he was involved in another breast medical malpractice case, Mr. X's. It was obvious to me that Dr. Loh had a history of withholding important diagnostic information, incorrectly diagnosing and treating breast conditions, and no one was stopping him from repeated offenses.

On a late March night in 2005, in frustrated emotions, I noticed I had spent the evening and late into the night emptying out my distraught emotions into type. My weak surgical right arm ached from all the typing At least I was tired now, so I crawled into bed. The night of wrath darkened my bedroom. It might have blinded me completely if it were not for the illuminating light of my sons sleeping peacefully nearby, awaking me to my need as I tried to shake off my angry darkness.

Chapter Learning Tips

The following list of suggestions may be helpful to those who may be preparing for and going to deposition:

1. Before deposition make sure you are prepared by reviewing the evidence of your misdiagnosis in your head so that you will be prepared to discuss these events.

2. Before deposition also arrange for any childcare that is needed, as it may be best not to take children with you to deposition.

3. You may want to take a friend with you to deposition for support.

4. Have the questions at deposition repeated, if you do not understand what is asked at deposition.

5. Try to be as accurate as possible and honest in all of your responses at deposition.

6. If you do not recall something that has been asked during deposition, just say you do not recall and be honest.

7. Take food and/or drinks with you to deposition, as deposition may be long.

8. Ask for breaks and bathroom use if deposition is long.

9. Sometime after deposition, ask for the deposition transcripts and read them over, noting any discrepancies between what you have reported and what your negligent doctor(s) have reported.

10. Prepare for trial by being confident in yourself and making sure your lawyer is prepared.

Chapter 7

Emotional/Spiritual Healings

Unwise people don't learn from their mistakes and often don't admit to their mistakes, smart people learn from their mistakes, and wise people learn from the mistakes of others.

-Robin Gray, March 1, 2005

The days were growing slightly warmer and longer, melting snow on the white-patched mountain near my home in April 2005. The seemingly perpetual, gray skies of winter were gradually fading, and rays of bright spring light projected from high to the worn, dormant tree limbs below, tantalizing hope and new life. It was due season for healing and rebirth

As I peered out my kitchen window frame bars, flushed while sipping a cup of hot green tea, I was irritated by the apparent changing of the seasons. I did not care much for the coming spring of April. I had grown accustomed to fighting the sterile, harsh, coldness of winter, keeping to myself, and writing with bitterness toward the physicians who misdiagnosed me. However, as I looked down at myself, I realized maybe I had become a little melancholy and cold in the process, not knowing it, and needed the sun's healing light.

As God's light reflected upon me through my son, Neo, who prayed and led me into biblical scripture, I miraculously desired a transformation of peace and tranquility. I no longer wanted to assume the role of the victim, but wanted to devote more time and energy into turning my adversities into light for others and to accepting my physicians' errors without anger.

I was led to pray several times a day for self-healing. As I prayed, I felt less depressed, and I felt compelled to put myself in the position of my incompetent physicians, who were in denial. I imagined how very difficult it might be to realize that your medical negligence had done harm to a patient, much less a colleague's spouse. Certainly, my physicians had the knowledge and skill to make a right diagnosis, but failed, which was obviously a horrible mistake for all parties. Perhaps icy, cold emotional distancing, not admitting their errors to me, was the only way they could cope with their mistakes. Such denial of faults and lack of self-monitoring was clearly wrong, but it was a means to their end.

I prayed for God to magically erase my misdiagnosis, not just for me but for everyone involved. However, nothing happened. I was disappointed, thinking I did not deserve everything that had gone so wrong.

Nonetheless, in the midst of my disappointments, I thanked God for allowing me to have my lump taken prior to an advanced cancer stage of no return. Additionally, I thanked God that the bulk of the tumor was a precancerous rather than an invasive cancer, as I surely would have had an extremely advanced cancer stage, if I were even alive at all.

Throughout my odd mix of disappointment and thankfulness I continued to meditate on Psalm 37:21 from the <u>King James Version Bible</u>, *"The wicked borroweth, and payeth not again: but the righteous showeth mercy, and giveth."* After repeatedly reading this scripture verse over the course of several weeks, with much difficulty and prayer, I finally managed to give up some of my anger over my physicians' inexplicable denial of medical mistakes. As a result, I felt a little more in control of my life and a bit more peaceful.

However, all that changed in November of 2005, when huge survival advantages of a new drug for early stage HER2 breast cancer were published in the New England Journal of Medicine. Immediately, I worried if I should have the newly approved early-stage breast cancer drug which was previously only available via clinical trial, so I researched Herceptin extensively.

Eventually, I found an expert oncologist in the HER2 pathways. He recommended that slices from my invasive breast cancer tissue block be retested for HER2 and pre-clinical molecular markers. When the tests results came back, they indicated that I was definitely HER2 positive and that I would respond, at least pre-clinically, to Herceptin. As a result, the expert oncologist recommended that I take nine weeks of late adjuvant Herceptin.

Anxious to prevent a HER2 breast cancer relapse, which is very aggressive and difficult to treat, I began intravenous Herceptin infusions about a week before my trial date. Of course, I was worried how I would do the therapy and go through trial.

Fortunately, a pre-trial settlement was offered to me only days before my trial in Jan. 2006 by both Dr. Loh and Dr. Lyon. I was very relieved and thankful that they were willing to settle, especially since I was getting intravenous Herceptin treatment.

However, the settlement amount offered was only marginally satisfying. This was especially true when that amount was reduced by about 30 percent after expenses and pre-set attorney contingency fees were accounted for.

Attorney Rich truly did become a partner to me. It seemed like I was hardly compensated for all that I had suffered. Nonetheless, I figured that nobody could ever pay enough for a delayed cancer diagnosis. Only the reversal of time with early diagnosis would ever truly be satisfying. Therefore, I agreed to the undisclosed settlement amount, knowing that at least I had made my negligent physicians accountable for their errors.

A few days after I settled on the phone with my attorney, I got the settlement document in the mail. I was shocked that the formal written settlement offer included stipulations and conditions that Attorney Rich had not warned me of when I accepted settlement. In particular, the settlement offer stated that not only did the physicians not admit to error, but they also demanded that all parties would not contact or communicate in any way regarding any and all issues relating to the lawsuit. To make matters worse, when I phoned Attorney Rich about the stipulations and tried to change them, I was informed it was too late to reverse things or go to trial.

At least Attorney Rich was apologetic about his failure to give me full disclosure of the settlement agreement. Still, I felt deflated like a popped balloon because I had always wanted to confront my physicians in hopes that they would admit their errors to me and apologize. However, those healing doors were now eternally shut, not by my will, but theirs.

I thought about their communication restrictions with sadness for a long time until I spoke to my mother who conveyed that it was their loss, not mine. As she put it, with their prior denials, they would never be able to admit the truth or offer any kindness. My husband may have stated the case even better, "Why want any communication with those who have done so much wrong without sorrow, acting like devils?" Put that way, I agreed that I did not want anything to do with those in darkness.

As the weeks passed, not surprisingly, my husband and I failed to hear any late apologies from my negligent physicians. A few times Isaac awkwardly ran into them at the hospital, but no apologies were offered. Several months passed and still no regrets were given, so Isaac finally took a nonverbal stand for the injustice that happened to me by writing both Dr. Loh and Dr, Lyon a letter of his disapproval and dissatisfaction, which seemed to help him put the whole ordeal out of his head.

As for me, I had a harder time trying to move forward with my misdiagnosis, especially since my negligent physicians denied any wrong doing. I was angry that they never apologized, even after the lawsuit, and that one of them continued to practice direct patient medical care. Knowing what they had done, I felt upset, as I tried to bury my emotions by keeping busy with my children and journalizing.

However, I had a hard time burying the pain my negligent, self-protecting physicians caused. Therefore, I read several Christian and self-help books on healing emotional pain, which helped me to put away some of my grudges and hurt feelings. The books made me realize that holding onto emotional pain only blocked me from healing, kept me physically and emotionally exhausted, and kept me from experiencing other positive blessings in life.

Acceptance has not been a one time act for me, but is something that I am challenged to do over and over again, being plagued with residual pain caused from many surgeries and treatments related to my misdiagnosis. Being human, in the midst of my pain, there are moments where anger desires to have the victory with me. However, those are the moments that I quickly reject anger and seek humble acceptance, so I will not be cheated out of blessings, peace, and other good things available in life.

I have found in the act of acceptance, a light that leads me out of the dark things that happened to me and into God's love, where there is life. I now realize that in order to gain life, sometimes you have to lose it. I had to lose my breast, lose some of the nerves in my arm from the lymph node dissection, temporarily lose my hair, and lose my ovarian hormones in order to save my life. Ironically, also losing yet another piece of me, my angry over my misdiagnosis and the aftermath, gives me back my life once again.

Now, as I live in humble acceptance, I have found blessings. I feel more calm and able to fully appreciate the beauty in life, while not focusing on negative things. In acceptance, I live more fully in God/Christ where there is love, totally void of anger and full of acceptance, humility, and forgiveness, the ability let go of the past. Miraculously, in Christ and humility, I have been lead to new doors where I find understanding and peace. In the doors of peace, I have discovered real life where I am more often able to live life in the moment and enjoy it, without being distracted by negative thoughts. I doubt that I would have found the pathway to peace via acceptance at such a young age, if it were not for my cancer experiences.

Today, I am extremely happy and grateful to say that I remain cancer free, while living in peaceful serenity and finding new doors of pleasure. I am pleased that I have had the opportunity to see my sons grow, and I have enjoyed passing onto them some of my talents, including writing, playing the clarinet and piano, and cooking. I also have had a wonderful time educating my youngest son at home for some of his school years. Had it not been for surviving cancer, I do not think I would have had the courage to instruct him at home or had the courage to write a book.

Hopefully for those who have already suffered a misdiagnosis, cancer diagnosis, or have suffered from life's inherent challenges, you also will find peace, acceptance, and new doors of life and opportunities. Discovery of acceptance and contentment, whatever your circumstance is, is a blessing. On the other hand, non-acceptance often only brings pain and suffering.

Now, for those misdiagnosed, let me stress acceptance of a misdiagnosis and moving forward does not mean that your negligent physicians should be let off the hook without responsibility. Negligent physicians need to be held accountable by being reported to their state's health department and/or being litigated. I highly recommend litigation for two reasons. First, it offers a chance for a patient to retrieve some of the financial loses that their negligent physician(s) have caused. Secondly, it may help improve patient care for others. For example, since my lawsuit settlement, both of my physicians have a record on their state's Health Department Doctor Profile website, which reflects that they each have made a malpractice settlement that is "relevant for patient decision making." I feel good knowing that other patients have access to this significant information, making them more informed health care consumers.

Although litigation may offer much, I must stress to those litigating that I believe that winning a malpractice lawsuit is far less important than finding acceptance and peace. Again, in finding acceptance, I have found new doors of happiness, life, and the ability to help others.

In an attempt to warn and to assist others, I have elaborated extensively on various unsuspected physician errors. However, I do not want to leave anyone with the impression that all physicians are bad. Many physicians are very competent and caring.

In fact, I had the pleasure of receiving care from one of the most outstanding breast surgeons in the world, the late Dr. Jeanne A. Petrek. I am thankful that I had her as my breast surgeon after I had been misdiagnosed with fibrocystic breast disease for nearly two years by Dr. Loh. Unlike Dr. Loh, who only mentioned a mastectomy as a surgical option to follow my lumpectomy, Dr. Petrek insisted on aggressive treatment with a mastectomy and sentinel node dissection. During the mastectomy, Dr. Petrek discovered more cancer just beyond the breast and removed it. I sincerely doubt that Dr. Loh would have discovered this remote area of cancer in my breast. Nor would he have discovered the cancer in my axillary lymph nodes since he did not even recommend a lymph node dissection surgery. Of course, the discovery of cancer in the lymph node necessitated chemotherapy, which I ultimately did receive. However, had I listened to Dr. Loh, I would have never known of the contaminated first lymph node or the need for further treatment with chemotherapy. I am convinced that I am here today, enjoying my family and friends, because of Dr. Petrek's expertise and aggressive treatment.

Dr. Petrek was more than an outstanding surgeon. She was also a fabulously compassionate patient advocate. Despite her busy schedule, she always answered not only every question that I had, but she also wanted to know how I was coping with everything. It was not unusual for her to call me several times, sacrificially on her own time during the weekends, to update me on my case and inform me of the necessary treatments required to eradicate my cancer.

Regrettably, not all physicians are as meticulous and compassionate. As you have seen, very capable doctors make devastating medical errors in breast assessment. Therefore, I have included a postscript following this chapter, which discusses how to help prevent a breast misdiagnosis.

Chapter Learning Tips

At some point you need to put your cancer diagnosis and/or misdiagnosis behind you and move forward. The following list may help you get a start to getting on with your life.

1. Enjoy the now and stay in the moment, without focusing too much on the past or future. Make a new life with new goals, which will make you feel better and more in control.

2. Think positive, putting things you can not change behind you.

3. Let the little stuff go and live more carefree.

4. Live a healthier and greener lifestyle. When you eat healthy and exercise, you feel better. Avoid high sugar content foods, high-fat foods, and make sure you eat many anti-oxidant foods like crustaceous vegetables, grapes, blueberries, and so on. Foods rich in vitamin D may also be helpful and have been found to help decrease certain breast cancer subtype relapses.

Postscript

Guide to Help Prevent a Breast Cancer Misdiagnosis

During the last few years, following my misdiagnosis, I have learned some shocking facts about the misdiagnosis of breast cancer. It is the most prevalent medical misdiagnosis in the United States, resulting in the most popular type of medical malpractice claim against physicians. (2) At least 10,000 women per year are victimized by a breast cancer misdiagnosis and outrageously most of these women are young. (3) In fact, younger women who are less than forty-five years of age with a self-discovered breast mass along with a negative mammogram account for over two thirds of patients sustaining a breast cancer misdiagnosis or delayed diagnosis. (4) This suggests that physicians may assume a lower cancer risk and do not aggressively rule out cancer in young women who have a negative mammogram and find their own masses. Often only a clinical breast exam, with or without mammography, is done with assurance that a breast lump is benign without the necessary breast biopsy, which is the leading cause of misdiagnosis. (5)

Unfortunately, physicians often misdiagnose young women with breast lumps for prolonged periods, with the average delay at about sixteen months, according to the recent 2002 Physician Insurers Association of America Study. (6) This is more than ample time to result in cancer progression with devastating results, including worse prognosis with more surgeries and treatments.

Despite the tragedy of a breast cancer misdiagnosis, it is a common misdiagnosis that has been occurring at an alarming rate in young women for many years. (7) In fact, it has been occurring since the early1900s, but it seems nobody knows about it. (8) The dirty secret is kept well hidden, as most breast malpractice cases are settled quietly. Furthermore, national health societies have not loudly announced that breast cancer misdiagnosis is frequent in young women. Instead, the only pubic message loudly heard is that all adult women should to do monthly self-breast exams, should start yearly mammograms at age forty, and should see their doctor immediately if a lump is found.

However, my motto is that once a breast lump or lumps are found, it is not enough to just see your physician. Instead, you must become your own advocate. Specifically, you must seek out the best medical care possible, and avoid the usual pitfalls that lead to a breast cancer misdiagnosis.

Of course, the best time to be vigilant about seeking accurate breast diagnosis is from the start. Survival increases with early diagnosis. Additionally, getting the correct diagnosis initially is vital, as correcting a wrong diagnosis at a later point is very difficult. This is because the mindset of the patient and doctor are already set, and changes to first impressions are unlikely or difficult. Therefore, it is essential to set out on the right course for breast assessment and diagnosis.

First, it is very important to choose the right physician sub-specialty for breast assessment. You probably will see your primary doctor, family doctor, or gynecologist first for a breast lump. These doctors will probably recommend you to see an experienced breast surgeon. Of course you can request a referral to a breast surgeon specialist, if a referral was not offered.

A breast surgeon preferable, as he/she is most qualified when a surgical breast biopsy or breast surgery is recommended or desired for a more definitive diagnosis.

You certainly need to be careful about checking the work records of your surgeon and any other physicians, such as radiologists and pathologists, involved with your breast care. First, make sure your physicians are licensed to practice medicine by checking with the state health department. Secondly, make sure your physicians are board certified in their specialty. Also, you may ask your friends, family, local hospitals, and other healthcare professionals about your physicians' work histories. If you dare, you can also ask your doctors if they have ever misdiagnosed breast cancer. However, most physicians will not divulge bad records. Therefore, you may want to check the health department where your physicians practice for negligence. For example, in New York, the Health Department has a Physician Profile website and an Office of Physician Medical Conduct website, which lists physician negligence and misconduct. However, be aware that these state health department websites do not always list all cases of physician medical malpractice. For more complete records of medical malpractice and summons and complaints, visit the county/city clerk's office in the town/city in which your physicians practice.

In addition, check to make sure your physicians have experience in breast assessment. Personally, I would make sure my doctors have at least five to ten years of experience in breast assessment and see hundreds of breast cases per year. Remember, larger cities and cancer centers have physicians with the most expertise in breast assessment. With something as important as your life, you may very well need to go out of your region to obtain the best breast care possible

Even when you have obtained excellent physician referrals and your doctors seem to have all the right experience and credentials, there may be times when you may need to fire your doctors and look for better doctors. This is particularly true if there are signs of cavalier physician behavior or signs of negligent behavior such as the following:

- You are told not to worry about your breast lump because a lot of young women have benign fibrocystic condition, benign fibroadenomas, or any other kind of benign lump.
- You are told you are too young for breast cancer. (Young women do get breast cancer!)
- You are told not to worry about your breast lump because your mammogram was normal. (Mammography, especially in younger women, cannot fully rule out breast.)
- You are told not to worry because your breast lump does not feel or look cancerous by physical exam. (The physical exam is subjective and can not completely rule out cancer.)
- The surgeon fails to take adequate breast, female, and family history. (Ideally, your physician should ask you about your breast-feeding history, any breast appearance changes, any nipple drainage, any past hormonal medication use, any radiation exposure to your chest, any pregnancies, and family history of breast cancer, especially earlier in life.)

- You feel rushed and hurried by the physician, or you are not allowed to fully explain your symptoms and breast history.

- The physician refuses, defers, or discourages your request or mention of a second opinion.

Second medical opinions should be encouraged by your doctor and will help reduce the chance of a misdiagnosis. In order to obtain an unbiased fresh diagnosis, it is wise not to inform the successive physician of the previous physician's diagnosis or recommendations. However, sometimes even second physician opinions are wrong, particularly when physicians over-rely on noninvasive diagnostic tests that cannot fully rule out breast cancer.

The only diagnostic test to determine the exact histological nature of a breast mass/lump is a representative biopsy that is properly read via microscopic examination. Notice I did say correctly read and correctly obtained! That's right, inadequate tissue biopsy sampling and misread pathologies do occur and can cause a breast cancer misdiagnosis.

Biopsy sample errors can occur when the surgeon does not adequately biopsy a breast lump and has left out vital tissue for pathology analysis. Both benign and cancerous lumps can coexist, which may increase this type of error. Also, fine needle aspiration (FNA), may contribute to sampling errors, especially if only limited areas of a mass are needled and sampled and has an error rate reported in the literature 1% to 35 %. (9). The core biopsy may be safer in terms of sampling than the FNA since it samples a larger specimen, using a larger bore needle than the FNA. Additionally, the core biopsy is often easier for the pathologist to read than the small sample cytology of the FNA. However, even the core biopsy has a 2 percent error rate where diagnosis of cancer is missed. (10) A total excisional biopsy, where the entire lump is removed, may be even the safest in terms of reducing sampling errors.

However, all biopsy types may be subject to biopsy pathology reading errors by the pathologist, even very rarely, the excisional biopsy. Pathology errors may be due to false negative or false positive pathology reports. You may be under-diagnosed or over-diagnosed in these instances. You may help reduce these types of errors by obtaining second opinions on pathology. When a second opinion is sought, it is best to try to obtain a breast pathologist for the interpretation of breast pathology. Larger cancer centers often have breast pathologists who will give second opinions on slides. When you mail your slides out for a second opinion, if possible, do not forward the original pathology report with the specimen as that may bias the next pathologist's diagnosis. Pathologists may tend to agree with prior pathology reports, which could be dangerous in the case of a borderline diagnosis from benign to malignant. Sometimes even repeat biopsies and second opinions may be erroneous, as the diagnostic opinions of multiple pathologists may be erroneous. (Note that several pathologists did misread my lumpectomy breast slides.)

Remember, no matter what your physician calls your breast lump, you want to be sure that he/she has properly ruled out any chance of cancer and has not misdiagnosed you. Unfortunately, diagnostic opinions of doctors may be in error. Even second opinions may be in error, as happened in my story. Therefore, removal of a persistent lump may be safest, even if it was diagnosed as benign, as a wrong benign diagnosis may have been given.

In fact, according to Sandhya Pruthi, MD, breast chemoprevention researcher for the Mayo Clinic, if a breast **mass persists, excision (removal) is indicated**! (11) Unfortunately, many physicians are not aware of such safe recommendations. Removal should occur in a timely manner because as cancer increases in size over time, the chance for spread with a worse prognosis increases also. Remember that breast cancer can double in size quickly in young women because of premenopausal circulating growth hormones, estrogen and progesterone.

Knowledge truly is the key to making you a more powerful consumer, and this is particularly true in light of avoiding a breast misdiagnosis. Hopefully, you will heed well to my warnings and become your own patient advocate, taking control of your healthcare, which may very well determine the quality and length of your life. I have listed some causes of breast cancer misdiagnosis and summary steps that I believe will help women obtain correct breast diagnosis and decrease the risk of misdiagnosis.

Physician Causes Leading to Misdiagnosis of a Breast Lump

- Diagnosing a breast lump as benign without a biopsy. This is the leading cause of breast cancer misdiagnosis as noted in the subtitle on p. 23.
- Misread biopsy or fine needle aspiration pathology.
- Biopsy sampling errors where cancer is missed.
- Not taking younger patients seriously and making a premature benign diagnosis, without adequate diagnostic testing and aggressive assessments.

- Not taking patient discovered masses seriously.
- Failure to acknowledge suspicious breast symptoms such as red/brown nipple drainage and breast retraction.
- Failure to biopsy and or remove a persistent breast mass.
- Failure of physician to acknowledge or feel a breast mass.

Steps to Help Prevent a Breast Cancer Misdiagnosis

1. Make sure you see the right sub-specialist doctor, a board certified, experienced breast surgeon, who has an outstanding track record for breast assessment. Often some of the best breast surgeons are found at leading cancer centers.

2. Optimize your patient comprehension and communication with your doctor.
- Fully explain your breast concerns, symptoms, and relevant patient history to your physician. (To assist you with this task, complete Appendix A- Fact Sheet and you may give a copy of it to your physician.)

3. Even if your doctor tells you that your breast lump is a benign, you may ask/demand to verify that with a biopsy early-on.

- **Assurance that a breast lump is benign without a biopsy is the leading cause for breast cancer misdiagnosis as explained in chapter two**.

4. Make sure your diagnostic tests, like mammograms and biopsies, are read by physicians who are certified and experienced in breast assessment. Some of the best breast specialists are found at larger cancer centers.

5. Obtain and read written reports of all diagnostic tests, like mammograms and biopsies, to assure you have been given the correct diagnosis.
- Check to see if you have the right name and birth date on the documents.
- Do the written reports agree with the verbal diagnosis from your doctor(s)?

6. Make sure you attend all follow-up appointments. Additionally, immediately discuss, in person with your surgeon, the results of diagnostic testing, rather than obtaining testing results over the telephone.
   .

7. Obtain second surgical opinions, if you wish to help decrease a chance of a breast misdiagnosis.
- Give your second opinion surgical doctor written copies of any diagnostic test results that you have had done, and try not telling

the second doctor of the first doctor's diagnosis, so that you get a fresh second opinion.

- Compare the opinions of the first and second doctor. Do the opinions of the first and second doctor match? Perhaps even a third medical opinion is necessary, if the first and second opinions do not match.

- If the opinions of your surgeons agree, a misdiagnosis MAY be reduced. Yes, second opinions, multiple diagnostic tests, and repeated diagnostic testing may reduce errors in diagnosis, but perhaps not always.

8. According to Sandhya Pruthi, MD, breast chemoprevention researcher for the Mayo Clinic, if a breast **mass persists, excision (removal) is indicated**! (12) Remember you may demand your physician to remove your breast lump, even if he or she believes it is benign, as diagnostic opinions and diagnostic tests may be subject to error.

Other Helpful Suggestions and Warnings

- Passing a triple test, which includes a benign biopsy report, benign physical breast exam, and benign mammogram/ultrasound, does not guarantee that a breast lump is benign, as often boasted. This is due to potential human errors in the interpretation of all test results.

- Second opinions on your lumpectomy and/or mastectomy pathology are sometimes vital to avoid a misdiagnosis. Should you obtain the wrong diagnosis, the surgical and medical oncology treatment will likely be wrong too, which could result in over or under treatment of your breast condition. When you obtain a second pathology opinion on your lumpectomy or mastectomy breast slides, make sure you have a pathologist specializing in breast pathology review them. You may have to mail your breast slides to a major cancer center where there is a breast pathologist.

Postscript

Appendix A- Patient Fact Sheet

<u>Current Breast History</u>

Date lump found.

Describe breast lump and involved breast

- Circle breast lump location-left or right breast

- Circle location of lump-lower or upper part of breast

- Circle location of lump-inner or outer aspect of breast\

- Circle location of lump-deep in breast or superficial

- Size of breast lump in inches or metric units:

- Is lump hard? Yes or No

- Circle lump mobility upon touch- movable or not movable

- Is lump is painful? Yes or NO

- Circle lump is round and smooth or it has edges and sides.

- Circle lump has breast dimpling or no dimpling.

- Any red/brown nipple drainage? Yes or NO

- Is there any nipple secretions at all when squeezed? Yes or NO

- Any spontaneous nipple secretions? Yes or No

- Are breasts symmetric or the same size? Yes or NO
- Any recent size changes in either breast? Yes or No-If yes, describe changes-

- Are there any other breast lumps? Yes or NO and where-

- Describe any other concerns:

Patient's Past History

- Any past breast lumps? Yes or No

- Any past breast problems? Yes or NO

- Any past breast biopsies? Yes or NO

- Any history of benign breast conditions? Yes or No

- Did you breast feed your children? Yes or NO

- Any other cancers that you had diagnosed? Yes or NO

Female History and Potential Risk Factors for Breast Cancer

- Date of any pregnancies, miscarriages or abortions.

- Birth control use? If yes, how long?

- Hormone replacement therapy use?

- Any other estrogen exposure use like DES?

- Smoking use. If yes, how long and how much?

- Alcohol use. If yes, how long and how much?

- Positive for breast cancer gene?

Family History Risk Factors

- Any breast cancer in siblings or mother?
-
- Any breast cancer in family before the age of forty?
-
- Any breast cancer gene carriers?
-
- Any ovarian and breast cancer combination in family?
-

Record and Date of Diagnostic Tests and Surgeries

1. Date of clinical breast exam, doctor visits and diagnosis type-

2. Date of mammogram and result-

3. Date of ultrasound of breast and result-

4. Date of breast biopsy and pathology result-

5. Date of any breast surgeries and pathology result-

Appendix B- Websites about Breast Lumps

American Cancer Society
http://www.cancer.org/docroot/NWS/content/NWS_1_1x_Physicians_May_D
elay_Breast_Cancer_Diagnosis.asp

Young Survival Coalition
www.youngsurvival.org

BreastCancer.Org
http://www.breastcancer.org/

Wrong Diagnosis
http://www.wrongdiagnosis.com/b/breast_cancer/malpractice.htm
This site offers case studies on wrong breast diagnoses.

Comprehensive Cancer Information - National Cancer Institute (NCI)
http://www.cancer.gov/

Dr. Susan Love Research Foundation
www.susanlovemd.com/

Susan G. Komen Breast Cancer Foundation
www.**komen**.org/

Second Opinion
Regional Cancer Foundation
http://thesecondopinion.org/

Two Minute Breast Exam
http://www.2minutebreastexam.com/

American Cancer Society Self Breast Exams
http://www.cancer.org/docroot/CRI/content/CRI_2_6x_How_to_perform_a_b
reast_self_exam_5.asp

Appendix C- Physicians' Main Errors

Chapter 1

Dr. Covington failed to inform me that I had a "category IV, suspicious for malignancy" mammogram report that was abnormal based on his physical exam. Nor did he ascertain that I have a written report of this vital information, which I only learned of after my misdiagnosis. Furthermore, Dr. Covington fail to tell me, as written in his report, that breast lump required a surgical biopsy if it did not resolve. Unfortunately, I only learned of the recommended biopsy several years later, after my misdiagnosis.

Dr. Loh had my mammogram report, but he also failed to inform me that Dr. Covington's report recommended a biopsy if my breast lump did not resolve and that the report was labeled "category IV, suspicious for malignancy" based on the physical exam. Instead, Dr. Loh erroneously informed me that my breast lump was **not** suspicious for malignancy and that it was fibrocystic breast condition and required no medical intervention. How outrageous, not only was my breast lump suspicious, as Dr. Covington documented in my mammogram report, but it was cancerous. Only a prompt representative surgical biopsy that was properly read would have revealed the malignancy early-on or perhaps an astute surgeon.

Chapter 2

In the three-week follow-up appointment, Dr. Loh continued to erroneously give me a benign fibrocystic diagnosis based only on another breast exam and my most recent breast history. Unfortunately, again he failed to do a breast biopsy, which was essential to help determine whether my breast lump was cancerous or not. Additionally, he steered me away from a second surgical opinion, assuring me that he was capable of caring for my breast lump.

At the four-month follow-up appointment, Dr. Loh continued to give me a fibrocystic diagnosis for my enlarging breast lump, after only doing a clinical breast exam and a fine needle aspiration. He neglected to tell me that the only way to assure a benign fibrocystic diagnosis is via a representative core or excisional biopsy, which is accurately read by a pathologist. As a result, Dr. Loh denied me the standard of care for full disclosure where accurate diagnostic options should have been disclosed to me. Additionally, he denied me proper standard of care, where in order to rule out cancer, the core or excisional biopsy should have been performed on my enlarging breast lump. Finally, Dr. Loh only made a delayed six-month follow-up visit with me, allowing my breast lump to grow larger.

In the meantime, Dr. Lyon misdiagnosed my March 2001 fine needle aspiration (FNA) as benign when it was cancerous. She not only failed to read the fine needle aspiration biopsy correctly, but she read them when they were cloudy and not adequate for evaluation.

When my six-month follow-up with Dr. Loh arrived in September of 2001, he continued to diagnose my much-enlarged lump as benign fibrocystic condition after only doing the clinical breast exam and breast ultrasound. He failed to do the necessary excisional biopsy for my persistent, suspicious, and enlarging breast lump. Sadly, Dr. Loh discharged me from further care in September 2001, stating that my breast lump was not suspicious for cancer and was only fibrocystic when the one-and-a-half-inch mass was cancerous.

Chapter 3

In April 2002, concerned that my breast lump was huge at two to three inches in diameter, I made an appointment with Dr. Loh. He did a repeat fine needle aspiration on my lump, failing to offer me or give me the safer core or excisional biopsy. Then even before he had my fine needle aspiration pathology result back, he inappropriately assured me that my breast lump was not suspicious and only fibrocystic. Finally, when I asked Dr. Loh if he was 100% sure of his diagnosis, he did not confess any uncertainty, but only stated that I could get a second opinion. Luckily, Dr. Cross, a local pathologist, diagnosed my 2002 fine needle aspiration slides as positive for breast cancer.

However, Dr. Cross diagnosed my 2002 breast lumpectomy pathology slides as only a precancerous, ductal carcinoma in situ (DCIS) with micro-invasion. However, in November 2003, multiple breast pathologists found that the area of micro-invasion was actually a small area of Her2 positive invasive breast cancer.

Chapter 4

After my 2002 lumpectomy breast slides were sent out for a second opinion, the group that received them allowed an anatomical pathologist, rather than a breast pathologist, to diagnose them. Unfortunately, the anatomical pathologist, like my local pathologist, misdiagnosed the lumpectomy slides as precancerous and my invasive cancer was not found until over a year later in Nov. 2003 via fourth and fifth breast pathology opinions.

Notes

1. Kern, "The delayed diagnosis of symptomatic breast cancer." 1598-1604.
2. Physicians Insurers Association of America (PIAA), *Breast Cancer Study. Third Edition*, 5.
3. Goodson, "Causes of physician delay in the diagnosis of breast cancer." 1343.
4. Kern, "The delayed diagnosis of symptomatic breast cancer." 1605.
5. Goodson, "Causes of physician delay in the diagnosis of breast cancer." 1343-1345.
6. Physicians Insurers Association of America (PIAA), *Breast Cancer Study. Third Edition,* 15.
7. Ibid., 5-7.
8. Kern, "The delayed diagnosis of symptomatic breast cancer." 1613.
9. Pruthi, "Detection and evaluation of a palpable breast mass."646.
10. Pruthi, "Detection and evaluation of a palpable breast mass."646.Kern,
11. Pruthi, "Detection and evaluation of a palpable breast mass."647.
12. Pruthi, "Detection and evaluation of a palpable breast mass."647.

Bibliography

1. Fox, G.P., Neilson, J.A. *Sue the Bastards*. Chicago, Illinois: NTC/Contemporary Publishing Group, Inc.; 1999: 55-72.
2. Goodson, William H. III, M.D., Moore, Dan H. II, M.D.. "Causes of physician delay in the diagnosis of breast cancer." *Arch Intern Med.* 2002: 1343-1348.
3. Harvey, Wachsman M.D., JD, Alschuler, Steven. *Lethal Medicine*. New York, New York: Henry Holt and Company, Inc.: 1993: 158.
4. Kern, Kenneth A., M.D.. "The delayed diagnosis of symptomatic breast cancer." In: Bland K.I., Copeland E.M. III, eds. *The Breast: Comprehensive Management of Benign and Malignant Disease. 2nd ed.* Philadelphia, Pa: WB Saunders Co.; 2004: 1588-1628.
5. Physicians Insurers Association of America (PIAA). *Breast Cancer Study. Third Edition.* Rockville, M.D.: PIAA; 2002: 1-34.
6. Pruthi Sandhya, M.D.. "Detection and evaluation of a palpable breast mass." *Mayo Clinic Proc.* 2001: 76:641-648..
7. Silva, Orlando E., M.D., and Zurrida, Stefano, M.D.. *Breast Cancer, A Practical Guide. 3rd ed.* Edinburgh, London, New York, Oxford, Philadelphia, St. Louis, Sydney, Toronto: Elsevier Limited; 2005: 3,565-584.

Author and Publisher Direct Quote Recognition and Appreciation

Chapter 1 and 2
Goodson, William H. III, M.D., Moore, Dan.H. II, M.D.. "Causes of physician delay in the diagnosis of breast cancer." *Arch Intern Med.* 2002: 1343-1348.

Chapter 3 and 6
Harvey, Wachsman, M.D., JD, Alschuler, Steven. *Lethal Medicine.* NewYork, New York: Henry Holt and Company, Inc.; 1993: 158.

Chapter 4
Silva, Orlando E., M.D. and Zurrida, Stefano, M.D.. *Breast Cancer, A Practical Guide. 3rd ed.* Edinburgh, London, New York, Oxford, Philadelphia, St. Louis, Sydney, Toronto: Elsevier Limited; 2005: 579.

Chapter 5
Logan, Gary. "Medical Updates-Second opinions needed." *Hopkins Medical News.* Winter 2001.

Glossary

adjuvant therapy -- Treatments like chemotherapy or radiation added after surgery that helps prevent a cancer relapse.

antiestrogen -- A drug that blocks the effects of estrogen in order to decrease a breast cancer relapse in hormonal positive, estrogen sensitive cancers.

atypical -- Not usual.

atypical hyperplasia -- Increased cellular proliferation with abnormal changes in the nucleus of cells, but not malignant.

axillary dissection -- A surgical procedure in which the lymph nodes in the armpit are removed and examined to find if cancer has spread beyond the breast.

benign -- Not cancerous or malignant.

biopsy -- A procedure in which bodily tissue/fluid samples are removed for microscopic examination to determine if cancer or abnormal cells are present.

breast implant -- An enclosed manmade sack that is filled with saline or silicone gel in order to create an artificial breast after a mastectomy. Also may be used for breast enhancement.

breast-self-exam (BSE) -- A technique done with the use of fingertips to check for lumps at the end of a menstrual cycle.

calcifications -- In mammography, tiny calcium deposits, possibly signifying cancerous changes.

chemotherapy -- A common breast cancer treatment where toxic drugs help destroy rapidly growing cancers.

core biopsy -- In this procedure, a large needle is placed into a mass/tumor and aspirated for biopsy tissue sample. The biopsy is usually sent to pathology for microscopic diagnosis.

cyst -- Refers to a fluid-filled sac; not solid.

cytology -- Microscopic study of cells that determines if cells are cancerous or benign.

ductal carcinoma in situ (DCIS) -- An early stage of cancer, in which the cancerous tumor is contained within the ducts and has not spread throughout the body, making it curable via surgery.

estrogen -- A female sex hormone produced primarily in the ovaries.

estrogen receptor assay -- A test to see if a breast tumor's cells grow in the presence of estrogen.

excisional biopsy -- A complete removal of a tumor/mass; sometimes called lumpectomy.

fibroadenoma -- An adenoma in the breast may feel hard and fibrous and is proven benign by an accurately read representative biopsy.

fibrocystic changes -- A misleading term that is used to describe certain benign changes in the breast; also called fibrocystic breast condition.

fine needle aspiration (FNA) or fine needle aspiration biopsy -- In this procedure, a tiny (fine) needle is placed into a mass, cyst or cysts so fluid or cells can be aspirated and possibly is sent to pathology for microscopic diagnosis.

hormone -- A chemical substance, such as estrogen or progesterone.

hormone receptor assay -- A test to see whether a breast tumor is affected by hormones like estrogen or progesterone.

hyperplasia -- A condition that refers to overabundance in the growth of cells, as in ductal hyperplasia.

immunocytochemistry -- A very sensitive pathology lab test used in sentinel lymph node evaluation to see if cancer is present and can reveal occult cancer and micrometastasis.

infiltrating ductal carcinoma -- A cancer that starts in the milk ducts of the breast and then breaks through the duct wall.

mammary lymph nodes -- Lymph nodes beneath the breast and axillary region.

lumpectomy -- Surgery to remove a mass/lump and a margin or small amount of surrounding normal tissue.

lymphedema -- Swelling that can be painful and persistent in the arm and is caused by breast surgery and lymph node removal.

mastectomy -- Surgery to remove all or part of the breast, including the nipple.

menopause -- The time when female monthly cycles of menstruation cease forever. Menopause usually occurs by age 51, but it can also be induced early by some chemotherapies and pelvic surgeries that destroy ovarian function.

metastasis -- The spread of cancer cells to distant areas of the body.

ovary -- Reproductive organ in the female pelvic region that makes estrogen.

palpation -- Using the fingertips to examine.

pathologist -- A physician who specializes in the microscopic examination of tissues/cells.

progesterone -- A female sex hormone released by the ovaries.

summons and complaint -- A written notification to a party named in a lawsuit directing the party to appear and defend or answer before an issuing court.

ultrasound -- An imaging procedure that uses sound waves and is a painless method to find out if a structure is solid or liquid.

www.ingramcontent.com/pod-product-compliance
Lightning Source LLC
Chambersburg PA
CBHW031202270326

41931CB00006B/370